THE FOG LIFTER

MAKING LIFE A BETTER PLACE TO LIVE

GARY BLACKFORD

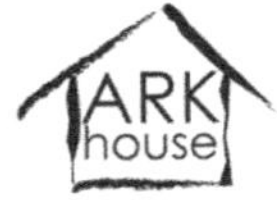

Ark House Press
PO Box 1722, Port Orchard, WA 98366 USA
PO Box 1321, Mona Vale NSW 1660 Australia
PO Box 318 334, West Harbour, Auckland 0661 New Zealand
arkhousepress.com

First printed 2012

Cataloguing in Publication Data:
Author: Blackford, Gary.
Title: The fog lifter / Gary Blackford.
ISBN: 9781921589720 (pbk.)
Subjects: Depressed persons--Australia--Biography.
Depression in men--Australia--Biography.
Dewey Number: 616.85270092

Cover design and layout by www.initiatemedia.net

ENDORSEMENTS

"Victor Frankel, once interred by Nazis in a concentration camp, reflected on his release that those who survived did so because they found hope for their futures. The Fog Lifter is a story of hope and offers a pathway and reasons for hope. With integrating personal experience and practical, biblical wisdom, this book will lead people through their journey, through the valley of the shadow of death, into a life beyond depression and mental illness."

Tony Sands, Pastor, 'Your Church' Church of Christ

'Gary writes with the authority of one who has grappled with the torment of mental anguish to emerge a champion leading other sufferers into personal victory out of their darkness. In this book, Gary identifies with readers in their inner struggles of confusion, depression, fear and panic, offering practical steps in the journey of total recovery. You'll be amazed by his up-close and personal insights, humored by his infectious candor and encouraged with his mix of empathy and strong love to rekindle the light of hope to live a purpose-filled life.'

Lorelle Magee, Pastor, Coffs Family Church

'Gary Blackford has been a friend and fellow minister here in Coffs Harbour for a number of years. As a pastor for over 14 years I am seeing an incredible rise in the numbers of people struggling with their emotional and mental health. Gary has written an outstanding book on depression and mental illness. It is full of real life experiences that will give hope to all readers, particularly those struggling in these areas. It's straightforward and easy to read, yet very powerful with practical examples to help readers biblically address some of their own issues. I highly recommend it to you.'

Shaun Foster, Pastor, C3 Church Coffs Harbour, NSW Director C3 Church International

'Gary's story of recovery is made even more inspiring by his desire to guide others out of the fog. The way through is presented in clear, practical steps, without discounting God's role in the healing process.'

Tony Colley, Cartoonist and Author

'Gary Blackford's easy-to-read testimony highlights God's overcoming power of release from the abyss of personal depression. It is not only challenging and frank but is an insightful handbook with some golden keys to freedom for anyone else caught in the grip of mental illness.'

Wayne Magee, President, The Foursquare Church Australia

CONTENTS

RAINDROPS KEEP FALLING ON MY—GOAT!

The sun was shining and the day was bright as I headed into my study to start to put into words the things running through my mind. The words were flowing as the keys took a pounding with my rather heavy two-finger typing style. It was truly a sight to behold as my fingers danced back and forth, rather like a cave troll swinging a heavy timber mallet across the keyboard.

There I was in my study, totally engrossed in the subject at hand, when all of a sudden a voice spoke from behind me, "Dad, do you think we should move the goat?" It was one of those random statements that you hear and then sort of wonder if you've heard right.

"What?" was my rather intellectual response, thinking the goat had tangled itself around something and become totally stuck. I really had no clue as to why my eldest daughter had appeared asking me about the goat.

She then said, "Well, Dad, it's pouring rain." As I swiveled on my chair to look out the window, sure enough it was. Besides the fact that the goat was getting rather wet, this instance reminded me of exactly why I'm writing this book.

On average, for one in four Australians, life can be just like that morning. You can suddenly go from feeling like you're walking in sunshine to cringing in the darkness of heavy clouds and rain. For many, it's perhaps more like what we call a 'pea souper', a fog that descends on mountainous areas, so thick that visibility beyond a few steps is impossible.

One of my favorite places is about an hour from our house. It's the charming little town of Dorrigo. This beautiful small country hamlet is situated on top of the escarpment at the edge of the Great Dividing Range. Dorrigo is surrounded by green lush fields and gentle rolling hills; it has dairy cows and beautiful forest areas complete with waterfalls, and is simply one of planet earth's special places. The main road is called The Waterfall Way, and it climbs the mountainside with breathtaking scenery at every turn. Yet, this stunning place gets some very thick 'pea souper' fogs. For some who read these pages, life has become a 'pea souper' fog that seems to have descended upon you and shrouded any beauty in a grey damp mist. How I hope these pages will begin to lift the fog for you and to blow away some misconceptions and wrong understandings so you can again see the beauty.

According to the *National Survey of Mental Illness and Well-being*[1], one in five Australians will suffer from mental illness during their life. More recent figures show that in the space of about a decade, around 25 percent of all Australians have either had in the past, are experiencing in the present, or will suffer from in the future, some sort of mental illness. These figures are based on reportable cases to a medical professional and do not include the millions of others who suffer from depression but who have never had it diagnosed. I read an article[2] recently that stated that since the global financial crisis hit, people seeking

---

1 National Survey of Mental Illness and Well-being. Australia 1997

2 Mental illness soars as global crisis hits By Jennifer Macey for "AM" Posted Mon May 4, 2009 9:32am AEST

medical advice relating to mental health has risen by 40 percent, and another article considers that at any given time up to 25 percent of the population is suffering with some sort of mental illness.

I wonder if 25 percent of our population suffered from any other particular illness, would not we as a nation be talking about it constantly, and trying with a great amount of effort to prevent or cure the sickness.

If this book has found its way into your hands, and you are one who suffers from some sort of depression or mental illness, then I welcome you to this journey, and thank you for the privilege of speaking into your life. I would ask you to consider the things you read carefully, and that you would grasp my heart in this, as one who has walked this very difficult road. In fact, in the first part of this book, I will tell a part of my personal journey through depression and mental illness.

Please do not expect a quick fix or a wave of a magic wand solution. However, do expect that there is a great hope for a better life. Let me be a life coach for you through this most challenging of subjects. What you experience today does not determine your future. There is a life full and free, where we are no longer bound to illness of the mind.

You are not alone on this journey. Try this—next time you are in a large group of people, whether in a shopping mall, large park area, or church, just stop and look for a moment. You can even start counting; one, two, three, and four. On four, think, 'Wow, that person today, or one of those four I just counted, could be suffering from depression or mental illness.' Do it again and again, and you start to get a sense of the numbers involved. The next time your mind tries to convince you that you're alone and no-one knows what you are going through, just remember to count to four. That's 25 percent of the population. You know the figures. Do the math. Probably the greatest error we make, and I have seen this many times, is to choose to isolate ourselves in our suffering. The problem is that we generally separate ourselves from the very people who can help us. We will look at this in depth later, but know this; if you suffer from depression or mental illness, you are not alone.

So this is how we will proceed:

I will give you a short journey through my life as a sufferer of depression and mental illness. This will include both before becoming a Christ follower, and also during my early years as a Christ follower.

I will go through some of the lessons I have learned along the way that relate to depression and mental illness, and how I can write these pages as a man who has walked this road and fought this fight, and who today can honestly say he is better for it.

In this book I will not be running through all the different types of mental and emotion-related illnesses, or try to define all the triggers associated with mental illness. For the sake of not being misunderstood, I will endeavor to use the descriptive terms 'depression' and 'mental illness' as generalizations, and cover a set of principles that will help all sufferers across the broad spectrum of mental and emotional issues.

These pages are not an attempt to write a thesis, or an attempt at an exploratory paper regarding the subject of depression and mental illness. My purpose in writing is to provide a story of hope. Just as, on one hand, hopelessness is extremely destructive, hope, on the other hand, is one of the most powerful forces in the universe. I desire through these pages to infuse in each one of us the hope for a better tomorrow. For sufferers, I want to give you a hope that the fog can lift and the days can become brighter, and an understanding that there *is* a place beyond the grasp of despair where the grip of depression is loosened.

Let me show you a way out of the fog, where we can look forward to tomorrow being a better day than today. To the carers, to give hope and comfort, and I pray, a pathway of hope through the maze of what can at times be an all consuming despair.

I attended a public forum on depression recently, and although it was very well-attended and the speakers were exceptional, I still found it lacking a very important piece of the puzzle. That piece is not just important, but rather vital for the understanding and treatment of depression and mental illness. In this forum, the only mention of the God perspective came in a derogatory way. For instance, a woman stood up to tell her story and she spoke extremely well, relating the story of her daughter who suffers from mental illness and telling of their challenges. It was a beautiful and heart touching story. What concerned me was that while her daughter was going through this very difficult time, she had the medical profession on one side advising medication for treatment. On the other side were what she termed the 'born again brethren' saying that the medical system is not to be trusted. The inference was that these supposed spiritual advisers were telling her that it's one or the other. I profoundly disagree with this misguided philosophy. I believe balance is the answer. I don't follow the humanistic 'purely medical problem' approach that throws drugs at everything it can with the philosophy of 'if it's purely a chemical imbalance, then the natural conclusion is that the cure must be purely chemical.' Nor do I hold to the 'purely spiritual' approach, which will inevitably lead to the conclusion that every problem comes from the sin nature, and therefore correction and repentance are the only answer. Both these philosophies have their elements of truth; however, taking any of these to an extreme is extremely dangerous. I will talk more about the quick fix mentality of modern day Christianity in a later chapter.

Let me assure you, before we head into my story, that God has a voice into this complicated and challenging human issue, and it is a voice of reason and of hope.

Certainly as a church leader, I would ask the question, "Why is it that depression, mental illness and emotional instabilities are rarely spoken of within our churches?" Some may consider that this does not affect a believer or Christ follower. I would profoundly disagree, as I see great numbers of people who genuinely love Jesus with their whole lives still suffering terribly through depression and other mental illnesses.

Mental illness is present within the church, just as it is within society. Many times it is masked and hidden, as thousands of people live lives crippled by guilt, shame and condemnation, afraid that they are not living for Christ as they should. Every time their mind disturbs them, more guilt is piled on until the person roams from church to church trying to genuinely seek for a solution. They are prayed for, expecting an instant miracle, and when they don't receive it, they go away in disappointment and sorrow, only to wander from one group to another, until their lives become shipwrecked in a never ending ocean of guilt and shame. Or worse, they forsake the pursuit of God all together and seek comfort amongst the myriad of false religions based upon works or connecting to some inner force of goodness.

I am aware that the painting I have placed before you is not a pretty picture. I just cannot stand the lack of understanding and misinterpretations that lead so many amazing people down a road of hurt and despair. These pages represent the greatest positive message of all. It is a message that can transform a life from being bound in the confines of depression and mental illness, to a life and mind set free and living beyond depression and mental illness. It is my hope and plan that everybody who reads this book, will come to an understanding that there is tremendous hope.

If you are reading these pages and you have never felt the bite of depression or mental illness in your life, I would hope that at least you would come to a greater understanding of those who do suffer in this way, and to hear God's voice in this issue. Chances are that every person turning these pages has suffered, or at least knows someone who suffers from depression or some sort of mental illness. Let us not just leave what needs to be said in the too hard basket. We need, for the sake of all who are going through these things, to get the truth into people's hands. These truths are the truths that will set us free. One of the things Jesus said while discussing how believers, and thus the church, should live is found in Matthew.

Matthew 25:34-36

> *I was hungry and you gave me something to eat, thirsty and you gave me something to drink. I was a stranger and you invited me in. I needed clothes and you clothed me. I was sick and you looked after me, I was in prison and you came to visit me.*

Let us not limit the 'sick' to those with physical illnesses, or those in 'prison' to steel bars of a cell. Thousands live a half-existence, emotionally and mentally sick, trapped in the prison of their minds and emotions. There is such a need for 'visiting' and 'caring' for these precious people.

Many people have used the following statement, and as a minister I have spoken on it many times over the years: '*He who the Son sets free, is free indeed.*' John 8:36 This verse is powerful, yet in my life, I quoted it and even preached sermons on it while still living in the reality of a mind that was not free. More on this later as we go through.

Just know this, as we head into my story, that there is such a place as life beyond depression and mental illness. I live there now. The road was not easy, but I am eternally grateful for the journey. So much so, that I would even say now how thankful I am for my mind. As you read my story, you will get an idea of how amazing it is that I can even say that. This mind of mine that I have hated passionately for many years turned out to be the very thing that led me to a place that is beyond depression and mental illness, and also to an understanding of God's grace and love that I don't think I would have had without this journey. I see now that the blackness can be the very thing that enhances the light.

My life has become so much better because of the journey. Life with its difficulties and trials has proved to have enhanced the life I now live. The fog has lifted, and the place I'm standing in is beautiful. Even if all you see today is the 'pea soup' fog around you, I ask you to walk with me through these pages. I am convinced that these principles will start to remove the clouds, lift the fog, and help you see beauty again.

WELCOME TO MY NIGHTMARE

"I can't go on like this. Why? What? I don't understand, or do I? No, not anymore. Why me, anyway? There's no use trying any more, I hate this, I hate it all, I hate me, and it's all fake. It's all wrong anyway, and it's so black."

Rounding a right hand curve in the road around 10pm, the place came into view. It was the part of the road that went close to the edge of the cliff. I had been there before. I knew the spot.

"It's OK, they'll all just think it was an accident. Mum and Dad will be fine after a while. I know they will be sad, but at least they won't really know." Still a fake until the end. The headline will read, "Young man driving too fast, loses control of car late at night." I will be just another statistic.

The car straightened as the speed increased. "So this is it, yeah, it's OK, they are better off without me."

How did it come to this? Why would a young man from a good home be only seconds from ending his own life?

One of the strange things about the subject we are covering in this book is that there really is no set formula for why it happens. From bipolar disorder to schizophrenia and depression there are some known triggers. However, being human as we are, the same stimuli can get opposite reactions from people who are in many other ways similar.

This is my story and yes, that was me in that car heading towards the cliff. Although it is obvious that I survived this attempt at suicide, I need to fill in some blanks on how I ended up on a lonely road in Sydney's south, accelerating a car toward the edge of a cliff.

I was a very sick child, a chronic asthmatic at a time when medication for asthma was in its infancy. As a young boy, I required large amounts of attention and if my parents were writing this book, 'large amounts' might just qualify as the understatement of the century. When I became mentally sick in my late teens and early twenties, I lost a large number of my childhood memories. I do however remember my mum and dad taking me from doctors to hospitals to special clinics for breathing techniques in the constant search for reasons and for help with my ill health. It may have been due to the large amount of medication that my immune system was so poor, because chest infections would regularly have me needing great care. My parents told me many years later that they spent hours awake just listening to me trying to breathe, wondering if I would last the night. As much as it shames me to say it, I was a 'high maintenance' child. I can almost hear my parents chuckling at this statement, saying, "Oh boy, you don't know the half of it!"

I do remember quite a happy childhood, apart from being sick, that is. I was the practical joker of the family, the type of child that would stick plastic spiders in my mom and dad's bed, pushing the spiders all the way to the bottom so their feet touched those nasty plastic creepy crawlies. I would hide in cupboards and jump out to frighten people. More than once I was sent away from the table for causing such laughter that rice would spray from mouths. I think at an early age I learnt to turn everything into a joke.

On one of my many days off school due to sickness (or in some cases, fake sickness) I was watching American daytime television (as if I wasn't sick enough already!) and the show *Donahue* came on. Donahue was the big star of American daytime television before Oprah Winfrey. On this particular day, he and his guest were talking about something called dyslexia, a word I had never heard of before. They started to describe the effects on reading and comprehension, with words moving, and the sufferer having to read over and over as the lines were jumbled. You guessed it, didn't you? Yes, I had that too. This did wonders for my already rather fragile self-esteem.

As you can imagine, educating me was, shall I say, a 'minor' challenge. Sorry, Mom! Actually, education was very difficult. I had an older sister and brother who were very good at school, so I ended up going to a different school from my siblings. Now I was not only the sick child and the high maintenance child but the dumb kid also. I didn't want to be at school so many times after taking the bus to school, I didn't go in or was only there for a very short time, if you know what I mean. School years were painful to say the least. I hated school, and school was not too fond of me either.

Being sick constantly was embarrassing. You remember the picking of sides for sport at school? The two captains stand opposite everyone else and start picking players. One picks one, then the other captain picks the next. I have heard stories of how humiliating it was to be picked last. Well, imagine this—I was always part of a duo and got picked with another kid, because the team knew that five minutes was about all I could play. "I'll have Gary.... (pause for effect that made me feel pretty small) and..."

I took great comfort in knowing that I must have been the ultimate 'super sub'. I played in the position of 'hooker'. To the unlearned about the football code known as Rugby League, played in Australia, this is the position in the centre of the scrum where a smaller person (namely me), has one huge guy on each side of him and another three big guys behind him, all packed into another group of people roughly the same size on the opposite team. The two smaller players in the middle are the 'hookers' who rake at the ball with their feet to win the possession. I loved it, but on a good day, about five minutes in, I was on the sideline wheezing with my inhaler, pumping medication into me and done for the match. Again, I take great comfort in knowing that for those five minutes on the field, the earth paused, as pure poetry in motion took the field. (I could go on and on, but it would only lead to more stretching of the truth!)

Leaving school as soon as possible, I started as a boilermaker's apprentice, amongst other jobs. It must have been around the age of 17 to19 that I started to develop some somewhat strange behavior. Things seemed to shift in a direction that would eventually lead me down a very dark tunnel. I still remember that tunnel and the consuming blackness; blackness so thick that it surrounded and overshadowed me. These bizarre changes around the late teenage years are not uncommon, and I have since found out that an alarming number of mental illness sufferers[3] begin to enter dangerous territory in their late teens.

Even today, I cannot tell you what triggered the shift or if it was sudden. I found I would spend hour after hour and day after day with hardly any sleep. I moved into a realm of living within my thoughts and finding some sort of comfort there, yet knowing all the time I was heading into dangerous water. I found the thoughts would run wild within my mind and I couldn't shut them off. Many times I didn't want to shut them off, as they gave me a bizarre sense of relief. I somehow knew things were getting worse and worse. My mind would race and race, going round and round as if it was being sucked into a giant vortex. I had one particularly frightening, recurring dream that would always leave me with a sense of riveting terror. Sometimes I kept myself awake for fear of having that dream again.

Hour after hour, I would sit awake at night lost in my thoughts. Unable to sleep, I would drive my car constantly. I'd drive into the city and through the notorious Kings Cross area

---

3 http://www.mindframe-media.info/site/index.cfm?display=85541

of Sydney at two or three o'clock in the morning. I would never get out of the car, I would just drive, lost in my thoughts. Other strange behaviors surfaced as well. For example, if there was a thunderstorm around, I would chase it by driving to where it seemed worst and stand out in it as if to say, "Come on, hit me." Or maybe it was just to sense the power, I don't really know.

If you've ever been white water rafting, this may serve as an illustration. There are rocks just under the surface and you're rolling from one to the next in turbulent water. Not being able to see what is just under the surface can be frightening enough, let alone the idea that you are being pushed along at an ever increasing speed, knowing at any moment you could tip and be lost. A current was taking me into black water and through caverns of my mind I could not fathom.

As the tunnel into which I was heading became darker, I would frequently self-medicate by consuming large amounts of alcohol. I found it to be the only way I could get some sound sleep. The boiler making didn't last and I started work in a bank. I found the bank a great place if you wished to be discipled in the fine art of alcohol consumption. Interesting that these are the people we entrust our money to. Any excuse was excuse enough for a drink. Lunch would be spent in the bar, as were the hours after work. Even our 15-minute break in the afternoon gave me just enough time to get from the fourth floor of Wales House in Sydney, down the elevator and across the road into the subway bar to throw down a beer and then be back at work. This was a regular part of life, or life as it had become. Often people I knew would find me asleep at the end of the bar, or the barman would wake me and send me home. There were no drunken brawls. I don't remember ever being an angry drunk, but I was a very sleepy one. At times I would wake up on trains facing the wrong direction. The train had been to the end of the line and was heading back on its return journey, as this semi-comatose, alcohol abusing, young person—me—slept on.

By the age of around 20, the blackness really began to consume me. I had developed what would later be described as paranoid schizophrenia. This became progressively worse to the point that each night I would check every part of my room and every part of each room on the level of the house I slept in. I would check under the beds and in all the cupboards, convinced that someone was going to be there. The strange thing is, that there was no reason for this behavior and there was certainly no logical reason that anyone would be waiting, hiding in my room to do me harm. After checking under, in, and around every part of my room, I would sit on my bed for hour after hour in a cold sweat, writing some very strange poetry, visualizing (or some may say hallucinating) as I wrote them. Sensing some sort of presence very close to me, yet feeling utterly alone, this seemingly tangible fear would grip and hold me in a place where I could not sleep.

Reason had left, or perhaps I had left reason, as my mind seemed to race faster and faster. I knew I was in trouble. When you write these sorts of things you cannot help but know. Knowing you're in trouble and seeing a way through are two very different things.

The poem below was written during one of those many fitful nights.

The Number 6?

'I walk the depth of hell',

I sort the meek from strong.

For only God knows how long,

How long indeed?

The question 'How long?' Oh yes,

How long. I must know!

It's this life or go. Yes,

This is it, it's no.6 'Oh to be a cat.'

Water from my eyes suddenly falls,

He's near me now.

Is this God or the devil?

I don't know. I don't understand.

Yes I do, it's just come to me,

This is a warning,

A warning to me.

My last chance, what will I do?

It's No.6 no more the fool.

No more time to just succumb,

I must be one, or what?

A feeling of deep despair has come over me.

Oh God help!!!

I-am-empty.

The next poem was written on a night where even now, some 25 years after I penned it, I still remember the dread of that night. These poems hopefully give you a sense of just how desolate and desperate I had become. I talk of 'blackness' rather than 'darkness' because this is how it felt.

West of Sydney are the Jenolan caves, a stunning cave system with beautiful stalactites, stalagmites and other amazing formations. I remember going there as a child. At one point the guide told everyone to stand still in the cave. To give us a sense of how dark it truly was, he turned off the lights. The blackness seemed to envelop us. It was so black that we literally couldn't see our hands in front of our faces.

My 'blackness' was something like that, yet blacker. It was an all consuming state that seemed to grab hold of me. There was something very much alive within the blackness, and although it's hard to explain, there was a very real evilness and sense of menace about it. In the caves the guide knew where the light switch was. The difference with me was that there was no switch to end my blackness, and that was terrifying.

On a night I will never forget I wrote these words while curled up in the fetal position on my bed in the early hours of the morning, unable to sleep and sweating a cold sweat as fear paralyzed me. A solitary street light from up the hill shone through the window. I was so confused and so caught within this situation, that I was actually living these words as I wrote them. I know it's hard to comprehend, but to my mind, every bit of it was totally real.

Walk with Me

'Through the dark forest,

Glancing at every tree.

Trees and more trees, I cannot see out,

Fell to my knees.

I look up ahead and

There in the mist

Stood a man,

My face clenched in his fist.

It is me, I'm sure of that, although slightly older perhaps.

Why? Is it a sign?

A gust of wind, the mist rolled away he was gone, and so to the day.

I must get back.

It's dark, quiet, the wind has died,

The mist is thick, it fills the night.

Ahead a light shone through the haze. I'm running, faster, faster,

Oh no!!!

He's back, beside the light,

Holding my face disappearing into the night.

I must see his face,

Who is this man?

He walks away, I start to follow.

I must know,

Obsession, yes, that's it.

Still walking closer, closer

Just a few steps separate us, will he stop?

Stop!!! I cried

But no response.

He walked, never turning to look

Never saying a word.

Up a track we walked,

The path was steep

The wind was strong,

I dare not speak.

The mist is thick, like mud I cannot see,

My arms reach out, my hands aren't free.

He stands before me.

His presence cold, the air freezes,

I feel ice, I feel snow.

Awake I cry, but alas no dream,

It was real, the man was me.

Twenty or more years later my eyes still fill with tears every time I read these words. We could have these words psychoanalyzed and discussed by great minds and I am sure that they would have thoughts and ideas as to the reasoning behind the grammatical variables, and as to why the tenses are at times messed up. I think the conclusion we would come up with, in layman's terms, is that at that time Gary was seriously messed up.

Some of my actions around that time prove that I knew I was in trouble. Around the age of 21 I worked for a home improvements company. I was a 'tin man', doing door to door sales of aluminum wall cladding. You might be thinking, 'how could such a messed up young person go door to door selling with a big smile on his face, and be doing quite well in the job?' That is a reasonable question, and the answer is this: I could fake it with the best of them. If you had known me at that time, you would have thought of Gary as a young man on the way up in the world. I had bought a sports car and had an attractive girlfriend. Outwardly I looked, for all intents and purposes, like a successful young man. This facade could not have been further from the truth.

I distinctly remember a moment that, in many ways, pushed me toward an eventual decision to take my own life. (This was about the same time I wrote the poem you just read called *Walk with Me*.) I pulled up in the driveway of a friend's house in the very nice part of Carlingford in Sydney's north west. As I got out my side, and my girlfriend got out the other side, my friend met us in the driveway. Walking towards us, he reached out his hand toward me and said a few words that cut me deeply. He said something to the effect of, "Man, you've really made it." I had the look, the stuff and the girl but when he said that, I knew what a lie I was living. Not that it stopped me from living that lie, but I knew, and I hated everything about me and who I was.

I knew I needed help and studying this later, I have discovered that some of my behavior was classic suicidal behavior. I remember leaving notes around my work office with drug addiction help numbers on them, hoping that a colleague would find them and offer me some sort of help. I didn't ever take drugs; I just knew I needed help. The bottle was my way of self-medicating. I know now I was getting more desperate inside, yet outside you could not tell.

Another episode that may show my crying out for help happened around the same time. I lay alone for hours on the floor of a house that four work associates lived in, until all my extremities went cold. Knowing that my workmates would come home sooner or later, find me, and try to help me, I continued to lie there. They came in late that evening and found me cold, in what they thought to be a semi-conscious state. They called the ambulance thinking I had collapsed physically but I had orchestrated the whole thing! I was just a young man who in some confused way, knew he needed help desperately.

I even called a Lifeline help number and told the lady I was going to kill myself. She was so nice and asked me to stay on the line while she got someone to help. I hung up! I've always wanted to, in some way, contact her, but I don't even know when I made the call. The poor lady has probably lived for years thinking I went and did it.

I know it sounds strange, but I desperately wanted help, but I didn't want anyone to know how messed up I was. Especially my family, who had put up with a sick, high maintenance, dumb person for such a long time. I just couldn't let them know that this facade of success was a lie, and the truth was that I really was just one big total failure.

A tangible fear had gripped my life. I feared living, I feared dying, I feared my facade being found out for what it was, and I feared people knowing the real, messed up me. I honestly don't know how to explain that fear. If you have or do suffer from it, you know what I mean. I am at a loss as to how to explain it if you've never lived there. It is a fear that never leaves you or sleeps, a fear that totally consumes your every waking hour!

These occurrences were not short term, and things continued to build up. Around 21 years of age, this 'got it all together', 'you've really made it', 'I wish I was more like you', young man made a decision. The decision would prove pivotal. The decision was to end my life.

My dad had two things we children were not allowed to have in our family as we grew up. These were firearms and motorbikes. I am eternally grateful for my father's stand on firearms, although I did get a motorbike later in my life, and I love them. I honestly think that if a firearm was easily available to me, I would have ended my life around then.

I planned to drive my car off a cliff near the old road around Heathcote in Sydney's south. This meant that everybody would think that I just lost control of my car late at night. I would have been an accident statistic rather than a suicide case. My mum and dad loved each other like crazy and still do. They loved us children in the same way, so I could not bring that pain on them. I left no note and didn't in any way showed them what I was planning. In a strange way, once the decision was made, I thought even more clearly.

The night I wrote *Walk with Me* was pivotal. It may have even been that same night that I decided to take my life, but I am not totally sure. I had what could only be described as a frightening spiritual vision or hallucination. You have to understand that by this time my mind was very close to melt-down. Visions and hallucinations were real and very much a part of my existence. The mind of someone suffering this way is anything but stable. Over a prolonged period, I had a few things happen that would be deemed as being in the very weird category.

Late one night as I sat shivering on my bed, after checking every conceivable space for this invisible predator who, my mind was convinced, was there, something very strange took place. I did question myself as to whether I would put this incident in this book. I think what swayed me to include it is that if this could happen to me, there may be someone who reads these pages that has had a similar thing happen. I remember the utter hopelessness of that night, and I guess I want anyone who can relate to this event to know that there is hope. To believe that there is no hope at all is to believe a lie. I believed it and I was wrong. Since then, I have learned that there is always hope, and I know just how powerful that hope can be. I know that to the sane mind this probably cannot be understood, and I'm okay with that. So, welcome to a confused mind's nightmare! It's the night the blackness consumed me.

The house we lived in was built in the seventies, and in my room there were three large floor-to-ceiling built-in wardrobe doors. They were all stained in that dark timber that was used a lot at that time. Something had drawn my eyes to stare at those doors, and what appeared on them was what I can only say to be a fuzziness of light. The light became brighter as I stared at this sight. I'm not sure for how long, but all of a sudden the light was seemingly overshadowed by this almost tangible darkness that not only filled the doors but seemed to also reach out and envelop my room in a sense of utter terror. It was so real that I curled up in the fetal position crying and shivering in fear. There was a presence in my room that night that was evil and I could not stop it. My mind had been taking me to dark places for a while now, yet this was a depth of despair and hopelessness I cannot with words come close to even describing. All was dark, I was lost, and all hope had gone.

Although I remember that night vividly and my eyes are full with tears as I write about it, the next part of my story is like a blur. I set my mind to finish with the pain and fear once and for all. I knew the cliff, I knew the place, and I set the day. That day I worked on selling and putting on the 'fake life', knowing what I was going to do on the way home.

Accelerating toward the cliff on that lonely road, on that very dark night, something happened. Whether it was actually audible or a voice in my mind, I believe that something spoke in that car as I pointed it toward the cliffs edge.

"There's something more."

These three words shot into my mind, although how I'm not totally sure. But they were enough for me to turn the wheel just before leaving the road that night. Stopped by the side of the road in confusion only meters from the cliff's edge, these three words were all I could think of.

"There's something more." But what?

I would like to say that I pulled the car over, knelt beside the road, asked Jesus to forgive all my sin, became a Christ follower that night and 'yeehah' I was rescued. This was not the case. I had been to Sunday school probably twice that I could remember. I had been engaged to a Catholic girl earlier on, and had to sit through those 'How to be a good Catholic' tapes. Within that process, I do distinctly remember saying to myself as I stopped listening to the tape: "if God is in this, I'm not interested in God."

I just couldn't see that I could live like I was anymore. I hated everything about myself; my constant sickness, being the family dummy and, most of all, being the fake I was. Oh yes, I was the 'life of the party' but I could not let anyone see the real me. However, those words "There's something more", would not leave me.

If there is a message I would like to take to this world full of people just like me, it's these words I somehow have from that night near that cliff, "There's something more", There is a reason to go on. Hopelessness is killing millions, yet there is a great hope for us all. I didn't know what that 'something more' was, and I am truly thankful that I had not been drinking that night, as I may not have even heard what was said.

Confusion reigned in me. The sleeplessness continued after hearing those words. The intensity and sometimes the strangeness of things increased. So vivid were these words, "There's something more", that after this suicide attempt I knew that there was something more, although I had no idea what it was. The fear still remained and my mind still raced and raced and I could not stop it. The thoughts and the nature of these thoughts were horrific.

I had a very strange thing happen at the Carlingford Catholic church. Driving late one night, as was my usual practice, I stopped outside the church building. Why that church? I had never been to a church meeting there, however my now ex-fiancée had taken me there to a youth group called Antioch a few times. So I guess it was a point of reference in some way. I had been to what they called an Antioch Weekend, where a group of youth spent the weekend at the church doing group things. I cannot remember what we did as, in all honesty, I went for the girls. I know... how shallow is that?

There was something nice about that weekend, and some of these people were genuinely happy people. On the Saturday night of the Antioch Weekend, something stirred in me, and if you wanted to, you could go and see the priest. This I did, and in that dimly lit room with candles, nothing really happened. That night came and went, and who knows if on that weekend I received something that helped me hear the "There's something more" I heard that fateful night.

The night I drove up to the church and something strange happened could have been weeks or months later. I parked on the street. It was late as I walked down to the church. I found the building open and there was not a soul around. Drawn by some urge, I walked in and sat down in the last pew facing toward the altar. (Here come the goose bumps. It happens every time I tell this.) I met someone that night and it wasn't just anyone. The church had a large timber altar at the front, and on the front of that altar was a small, simple empty cross. In the room were other very large and ornate crucifixes with images of Jesus on them, yet something was very different about this empty cross. As I sat there, I could not keep my eyes off that small plain timber cross. It seemed to brighten in the very dim room. Then a man appeared, I cannot tell you why, but what was amazing was that I knew who it was. I cannot remember his face or what he said, but something inside me knew him. There, alone in that dimly lit building, he came and sat next to me. I think for the first time since entering the dark caverns of the mind, I felt peace. I cannot tell you what he said, nor can I explain the way he vanished. But, all these years later, my memory can take me to that exact spot and I can see the shape of him in the darkness. In my memory I cannot see his face, yet I can still see him, this lone figure, walking down the center of the church as if he came from that single small cross to sit with me. Something inside me knew that he understood.

I do distinctly remember what I did next. Once he was gone, I ran out of the church building, jumped into my car and flew around to a person's house who I knew went to that church. This was a beautiful family who would have received the shock of their lives when late at night, a young 21 year-old man came knocking (rather loudly), on their door. When they opened the door, they were met by this statement: "I've just met Jesus."

As a pastor now, I would read this sort of thing and think 'Finally, he's become a Christian and all will be well.'

Not yet. Something did happen that night, and I believe with all my heart that Jesus showed up and met me there. However, life was still full of blackness, and although I had met hope for the first time, I was still well and truly lost.

You would think that someone who visibly meets Jesus would

be sorted out wouldn't you? Well I was still very messed up and obviously a bit thick as well. I was still awake all night lost in my thoughts and desperately confused. I would sink into a depressive episode incredibly quickly. I was still living the fake life and still hating everything about myself!

During this time, things seemed to move very fast and the pressure increased. I had a constant sense that something was about to happen, and it was like a foreboding that was ever present. My mind was something like a machine bearing that had run too fast for too long and under too much load. It was about to give way and burn out. It did burn out, and rather dramatically as well. The catalyst was probably when I smashed my car one afternoon. I don't think I drove that car again because after it was repaired, it ended up being re-possessed. Left with a loaner, an old Holden Kingswood from the smash repairers, something gave way, something snapped.

In an instant of despair, it all came tumbling down. My mind had run too fast for far too long, and it overloaded. My body had felt the effects of constant sleeplessness and tension for an extended period.

I stopped the car outside my parents' house in Carlingford. Why then, I don't know but I physically and mentally shut down. I don't know the technical term of what happened, and I cannot tell you how long I was there for. I don't know why I was able to get to my parents' house and no further. I do remember my father as he found me slumped over the wheel of the beat up old Kingswood, unable to move or really even communicate. It was as if my mind and body had simultaneously said, 'okay, enough' and stopped. I will never forget the love that man had, and still has, for his messed up son. I have a vague image in my mind of Dad opening the door of that car and reaching for me, but I don't think I could even respond. What followed was a blur of activity. I don't remember a lot of it, but it did involve hospital, lots of tests, doctors, and mental health professionals. My psychiatrist suggested I move away from Sydney for a time, simply to change the environment. After several appointments, I eventually broke into a sobbing mess. This was after being very angry with him, only because he didn't have a couch for me to lie on, and because he didn't sit beside me and say, "So when did all this begin?" It happened like that in the movies, why not for me?

Moving to Coffs Harbour on the beautiful north coast of New South Wales, I lived at the backpackers' and had my Honda VF motorbike. The sports car was repossessed after it was fixed, and I was not in a fit state to work or drive. Probably not even to ride a bike, but I did! Anyway, I would ride and ride my bike up and down the coast. It is so interesting how our coping mechanisms surface so quickly. I was away from Sydney, but I was not changed. I was working nights in a bar or at a resort, and generally getting involved with the wrong crowds. Sleep was still difficult and although I had stopped drinking alcohol, my mind would still race. I had so quickly switched into survival mode again. I was Mr Cool with the nice bike, long hair (I do miss the hair), and leathers.

When riding around Coffs Harbour to the north of the city, only a few hundred meters past the Big Banana, Coffs Harbour's most famous landmark, there is a church building with a blue cross on the roof that is lit up at night. Many trees cover most of the view from the highway now, but 20 or more years ago, you could see it clearly as you drove or rode down the highway.

Working as a barman in a resort close to that church building, I met a young girl on the staff who went there. She said it was pretty cool. The words 'church' and 'cool' had never really fit in the same sentence before but I was however convinced that there was something more, especially after my encounter with Jesus. So riding one Wednesday night, I ended up at this church building. I didn't know what to expect. They were having a church meeting when I arrived. My planned quiet entrance wasn't to be, as everyone knew I had arrived due not so much to the noise of the motorbike, but rather an overzealous sausage dog. This dog had little dog complex and thought it was an Alsatian, so it barked and barked at this leather clad unshaven biker. I stuck my head in the door as everybody turned around to look at what all the commotion was about. I met some beautiful people that night and they seemed to accept me, not that they really knew me. It was quite a relief that they were not all scary with two heads, just genuine real people. They even invited me to their house for supper. I was a stranger and they invited me in. How weird is that?

I ended up a short time later at a youth camp on the June long weekend in Tallebudgera, Gold Coast Queensland. I was about to have an encounter that would change my life forever! I was about to find out what that 'something more' was.

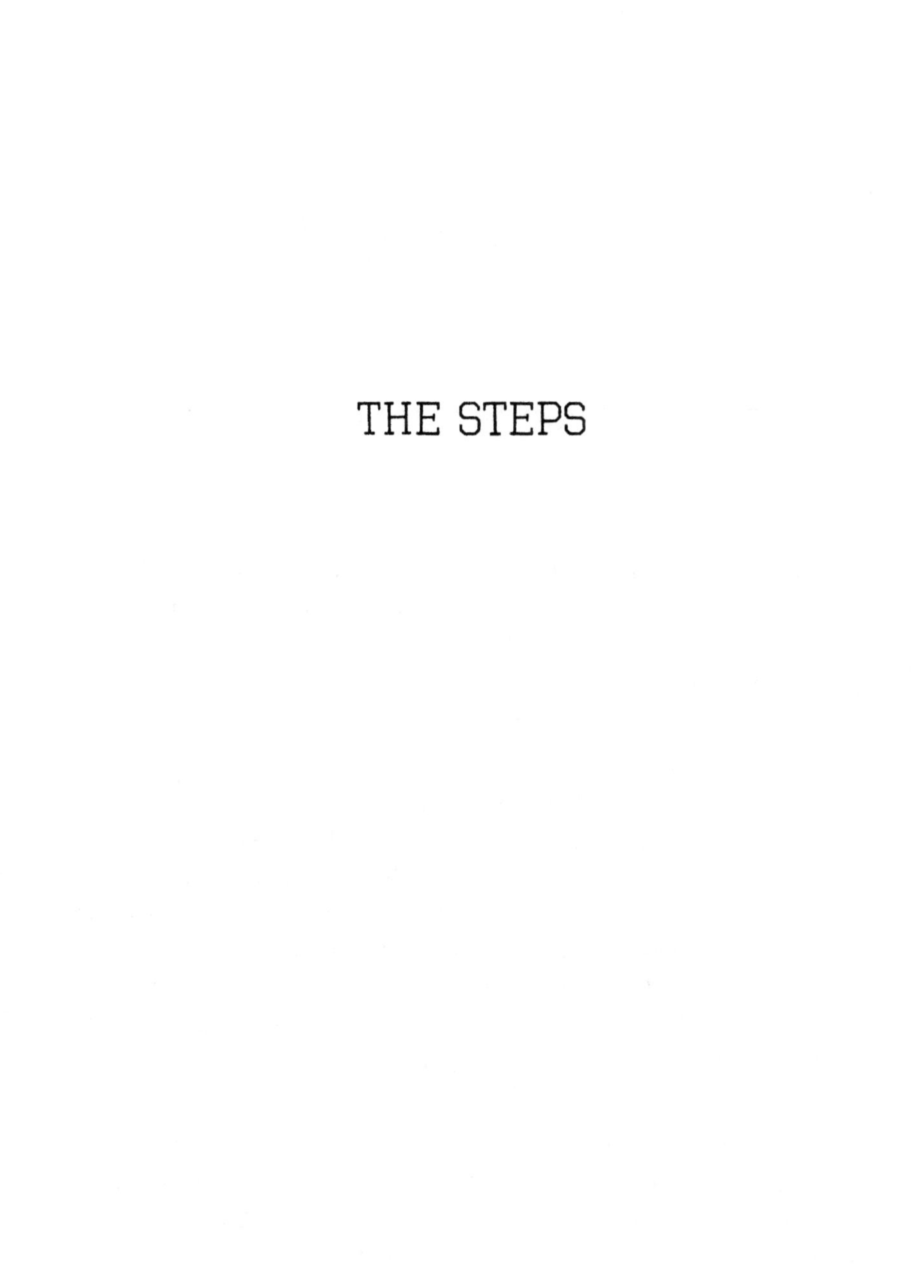

THE STEPS

METAMORPHOSIS OF THE MIND

STEP 1: BREAKING THE QUICK FIX MENTALITY

"I can't stand it," I said as I got up from my seat in an old hall filled with about 100 youth. It was a Saturday evening and I walked out feeling an intensifying physical pain gripping the area around my chest. This was not a normal sore chest pain from breathing heavily. This was different, in a strange way.

'I need to be in there!' was the thought that kept pounding within my mind as I made my way back inside that old hall. 'What is this pain? It keeps getting worse. I'm out of here.' Again I walked back out of the hall. Before long I went back inside, still in pain, yet needing to be in there. Five times during this youth meeting I walked out and four times I walked back in. The pain in my chest had reached the point of having me crippled and bent over as I stumbled towards the hall the final time but the meeting had finished, and as I tried to get back in, the crowd began to filter out.

So much pain gripped my chest that I was literally struggling to stand as I stumbled toward the hall. I spotted Phillip Bramble, who was the first person I had met that Wednesday night a few weeks earlier, when I arrived at the church to be greeted by an overzealous sausage dog welcoming committee. As I staggered toward him almost doubled over, I said something to the effect of, "I need help, Phil." Within a short time, I was sitting in a small room with another person who led me through a simple, yet amazing moment.

That night at a youth camp in Tallebudgera, Queensland, I became a Christ follower. I really didn't know what that meant. I prayed a very simple prayer and in an instant, many things changed. The first evidence that things were different now was that the intense chest pain that had come upon me was now gone. I said, "Amen," and it was gone. I cannot explain it, it was just gone, and I knew things would never be the same again.

That morning, a small group of us had gone to a local shopping mall to buy U2's latest album called *The Joshua Tree*. (Yes, that was the first time they released it.) My favorite song was *I Still Haven't Found What I'm Looking For*. Well, on that Saturday night I found what I was looking for! Not only had that intense pain instantly gone, but I knew several things. I'm really not sure how I knew them but I did.

I knew from that moment that I was loved by a God whose passion for me cannot be fathomed,

I knew He saw me in my darkness, and that He understood my pain. He not only understood, but chose to love me despite the disaster I was. The understanding that He saw me in all those dark places still astounds me today.

I knew in an instant that all my many mistakes were completely forgiven. I cannot explain why, I just knew.

Along with the chest pain vanishing, other things happened that day.

A peace flooded me, which I can only describe as supernatural. I remember the sleep I had that night. Or should I say, I don't remember that sleep, because it was the most peaceful sleep I could have ever had—it was awesome. I don't think I even dreamed. The best way to describe that night is 'restful'. My mind rested.

All the longing was turned to this amazing sense of happiness. Others on that camp say that I hugged everything in sight. Robyn, who would become my wife a few years later, said I even hugged her. I don't remember hugging her, and that's a tough one to live down—not remembering the first time you hugged your future wife!

My life was changed that night, and it's a night I will never forget. However, not everything changed instantly. My paranoid schizophrenia was dramatically altered and I never had to go checking under beds again. It would not be a stretch to say that the paranoia was instantly healed. The perfect love I met in the perfect Savior that night truly did drive out that fear. But my mind was still in need of a major renovation.

I firmly believe in instant healing; I have prayed for people and this has happened. Many things within me were instantly changed that day, and for this I am truly thankful.

I had spent about four to six years intensely mentally ill. I had walked a very dark road to reach this point and yes, the light of Christ did come upon me and change me dramatically. But in this chapter, I would like to show that while God does heal instantly in many cases, dealing with mental illness and the patterning of our minds is more of a process, rather than an instant fix. Although God had done something amazing within me, I was still sick. Now that may mess with some theology, but it's the truth nonetheless.

With depression and mental and emotional health issues, I find there is a tendency for people genuinely in need of healing to come to church and come forward for prayer in hope that their minds will be instantly transformed in a moment, and that they will walk away and never have a destructive thought again. It simply does not work that way, and creating that perception leads to many people just wandering from church to church, never getting healed and feeling even guiltier and more condemned than before.

I will be using many passages taken directly from the Bible that relate to health issues and their recovery, either from mental or physical illness.

Matthew 25:35, 36 (NLT)

For I was hungry, and you fed me. I was thirsty, and you gave me a drink. I was a stranger, and you invited me into your home. I was naked, and you gave me clothing. I was sick, and you cared for me. I was in prison, and you visited me.'

If it's all about quick fix healing, why then doesn't this passage say something like, 'I was sick and you prayed for me and I was well?' Again, healing is a reality and instant healing is a blessing, however it's the 'one size fits all', 'blab it and grab it' mentality I dislike. I tend to agree with the statement Martyn Lloyd Jones makes:

"Many Christian people in fact, are in utter ignorance concerning this realm where the borderlines between the physical, psychological and spiritual meet. Frequently I have found that such [church] leaders had treated those whose trouble was obviously mainly physical or psychological, in a purely spiritual manner; and if you do so, you not only don't help. You aggravate the problem."[4]

This statement is evidenced by the fruit it has produced. You can walk into any psychiatric ward around this country and most likely all of those locked in these wards, for their own and others' protection, will have had some sort of Christian experience involving prayer and sorrow. I have seen health professionals roll their eyes as a mental illness sufferer stands before them and says, "I've become a Christian now."

---

4 Martyn Lloyd Jones, The Christian Warfare (Grand Rapids: Baker, 1976), 206-208.

The health professional knows, because they have seen it many times, what is likely to happen. The person stops taking their medication and subsequently goes into a euphoric high, only to be followed by a crashing deep low. This low will be intense in its severity due to the instant ceasing of medication. Yet added to this and making it worse will be that this poor person's newly-found faith does not seem to have 'worked'.

Does this mean that Jesus does not heal, or even worse, He punishes some and heals others? No, of course not. Think of it like this: I have a friend who suffered from a physical disease and who went out for prayer every week. After nothing seemed to have happened instantly, he would presume that God had not touched him, and next week would try again.

The truth is, God had touched him and was in the process of healing. However, during this process of healing, my friend was learning his dietary boundaries. If God had waved His heavenly magic wand and healed him instantly, he would have never learned the valuable lessons he needed to learn to stay well. Where do we get the idea that we can treat our bodies in a wrong way and because God is a God of love and healing, come to Him expecting Him to fix the things that we should take action on ourselves? Our character development is more important to God than the speed of our physical healing.

I have learned this: God would much rather we are people of great character, even if it takes walking with a limp to get us there.

Think about this for a moment. Sometimes the greatest blessing a person can receive is not to receive an instant healing. I will say that again, and I know this can fly in the face of some people's theology; but it is truth nonetheless!

Sometimes the greatest blessing a person can receive is not to receive an instant healing.

If you have ever tried to renovate a house you will know that a renovation is never done instantly. It takes time. The book of Romans says this:

Romans 12:2

Do not conform any longer to the pattern of this world, but be transformed by the renewing of your mind. Then you will be able to test and approve what God's will is—his good, pleasing and perfect will.

The word 'transformed' in this verse comes from the Greek word *metamorphoo*, which is the same word we get metamorphosis from. 'Renewing' literally means 'renovation', or 'to bring about a complete change for the better'.

So we could read that verse like this:

'Do not conform any longer to the pattern of this world, but go through a metamorphosis or renovation to bring about a complete change for the better with your mind. Then you will be able to test and approve what God's will is.'

We need to see that healing from depression and mental illness is far more a process than something instant. It is however, a healing nonetheless!

Let's look for a moment at a few biblical examples of godly people who suffered from mental anguish.

MOSES

Moses went through some very difficult times in the desert years.

Numbers 11:11-15 (MSG)

Moses said to God, "Why are you treating me this way? What did I ever do to you to deserve this? Did I conceive them? Was I their mother? So why dump the responsibility of this people on me? Why tell me to carry them around like a nursing mother, carry them all the way to the land you promised to their ancestors?

Where am I supposed to get meat for all these people who are whining to me, 'Give us meat; we want meat.' I can't do this by myself—it's too much, all these people. If this is how you intend to treat me, do me a favor and kill me. I've seen enough; I've had enough. Let me out of here."

Numbers 11:14

I cannot carry all these people by myself; the burden is too heavy for me.

JONAH

Jonah suffered despondency to the point of despair.

Jonah 4:1-5 (MSG)

Jonah was furious. He lost his temper. He yelled at God, "God! I knew it—when I was back home, I knew this was going to happen! That's why I ran off to Tarshish! I knew you were sheer grace and mercy, not easily angered, rich in love, and ready at the drop of a hat to turn your plans of punishment into a program of forgiveness!

"So, God, if you won't kill them, kill me! I'm better off dead!"

God said, "What do you have to be angry about?"

But Jonah just left. He went out of the city to the east and sat down in a sulk. He put together a makeshift shelter of leafy branches and sat there in the shade to see what would happen to the city.

JOB

Reading the book of Job, we see Job suffering and battling with thoughts relentlessly through an extended time of difficulty and loss. Below are some examples of things he said while struggling with life.

Job 6:2-3

If only my anguish could be weighed and all my misery be placed on the scales! It would surely outweigh the sand of the seas—no wonder my words have been impetuous.

Job 7:11

Therefore I will not keep silent; I will speak out in the anguish of my spirit, I will complain in the bitterness of my soul.

THE PSALMIST

If the writer of Psalm 88 isn't experiencing misery of the soul I don't know who is. His words are those of someone extremely troubled.

Psalm 88:15

From my youth I have been afflicted and close to death; I have suffered your terrors and am in despair.

Psalm 88:15 (MSG)

"For as long as I remember I've been hurting; I've taken the worst you can hand out, and I've had it."

JEREMIAH

Like many Old Testament people who suffered from mental anguish, Jeremiah put his thoughts into verse, and we see this passage below showing a genuine bitterness of soul.

Jeremiah 20:14-18

Cursed be the day I was born! May the day my mother bore me not be blessed! Cursed be the man who brought my father the news, who made him very glad, saying, "A child is born to you—a son!" May that man be like the towns the LORD overthrew without pity. May he hear wailing in the morning, a battle cry at noon. For he did not kill me in the womb, with my mother as my grave, her womb enlarged forever. Why did I ever come out of the womb to see trouble and sorrow and to end my days in shame?

ELIJAH

The classic example is Elijah who, after a point of great victory in which he destroyed 450 false prophets and proved beyond a shadow of doubt that the Lord is God, still struggled emotionally. (Take some time to read the beginning of the story in 1 Kings 18 first.)

1 Kings 19:2

So Jezebel sent a messenger to Elijah to say, "May the gods deal with me, be it ever so severely, if by this time tomorrow I do not make your life like that of one of them."

The threat from Jezebel throws Elijah into total meltdown. This shows us that it can take but a moment to go from the sun shining, the roses blooming and rain falling in the desert with thousands returning to their God, to a man disappearing into the desert, wanting to die.

Look at verses 3 to 5 of chapter 19, and see the despair of this God-loving believer. 'I have had enough, Lord,' and 'Take my life, *I am no better than my ancestors*.' This was truly a broken man. His hope and dreams were shattered and his mind confused. He could only focus on the one point of trouble and that clouded out the thousands of people who had just come back to God with their lives changed positively.

The rain was falling again in the country that had been shattered by drought. Yet with all these positives, Elijah could not rise above the thoughts of despair and hopelessness under the intimidation of Jezebel. This is such an accurate picture of what so many of us go through in life. Elijah's recovery was not instantaneous. It took time to travel to where he needed to get help, and thankfully he traveled toward God and not away from Him, like so many do. It took time to sit and wait on God and time to listen and move out of his cave when God spoke. It took time to fulfil God's plans afterwards, and just as it took time for Elijah, it will take time for each one walking this road toward recovery.

KING DAVID

One of the things I personally love about David is his willingness to be real. He does not hold back about his failings and certainly does not try to make himself out to be some super spiritual guru. There is nothing more refreshing then people who are just real. One of my issues with many who follow Christ (and I have done it myself) is that we seem to think that we have to give the impression that we have it all worked out. David's honesty is great. He approaches God saying, "God, I'm messed up. Help!" How refreshing is that!

Psalm 6:2-7

Be merciful to me, LORD, for I am faint; O LORD, heal me, for my bones are in agony.

My soul is in anguish. How long, O LORD, how long?

Turn, O LORD, and deliver me; save me because of your unfailing love.

No one remembers you when he is dead. Who praises you from the grave?

I am worn out from groaning; all night long I flood my bed with weeping and drench my couch with tears.

My eyes grow weak with sorrow; they fail because of all my foes.

Psalm 13:2

How long must I wrestle with my thoughts and every day have sorrow in my heart? How long will my enemy triumph over me?

Psalm 18:4-6

The cords of death entangled me; the torrents of destruction overwhelmed me.

The cords of the grave coiled around me; the snares of death confronted me.

In my distress I called to the LORD; I cried to my God for help. From his temple he heard my voice; my cry came before him, into his ears.

Even in the much loved Psalm 23, David talks of walking 'through the valley of the shadow of death.'

Psalm 25:16-18

[Lord] turn to me and be gracious to me, for I am lonely and afflicted.

The troubles of my heart are multiplied; bring me out of my distresses.

Behold my affliction and my pain and forgive all my sins [of thinking and doing].

JESUS

Even in the case of Jesus, being '*sorrowful unto death*' Mark 14:34 (KJV), shows at least in part the mental and emotional suffering that Jesus went through. The Bible also states that Jesus was tempted in all ways and that He is touched with the feelings of our weaknesses. So it is clear that Jesus understands, and has suffered in some degree from mental anguish. Let us change how we think in relation to mental anguish and illness, and the work of God in our lives.

Ephesians 4:17

So I tell you this, and insist on it in the Lord, that you must no longer live as the Gentiles do, in the futility of their thinking.

I find it incredibly refreshing to have examples of real men willing to tell the world for centuries that they suffered so greatly. I can just imagine that somewhere in the wisdom of an endlessly wise God who knows the beginning from the end, He foresaw a time when depression and mental illness would be as prevalent as it is today in our society. I imagine that these words were written for us to read, to be encouraged by and through which to be given hope and, that in the mix of all our minds, is a loving heavenly Father helping and leading us through.

I need to cover the whole demon possession issue briefly. I have been in the presence of genuine evil several times. I experienced this before coming to Christ, in those dark and evil days.

In India, I have seen evil. On a trip to India I spent some time speaking to a family through an interpreter and I would say the mother was definitely under the influence of a demonic spirit. Her eyes were blackened and a sense of tangible darkness was present. It took a while to get through to them, and especially to the woman, but when it clicked and they asked Jesus into their lives and forsook their Hindu gods, the transformation was stunning. Her whole demeanor changed instantly and something like a black cloud left her eyes. The power of Christ visibly showed the darkness who the boss was. I will never forget the way her face lit up. These cases are real and evident, showing the power of Christ over the evil one.

I stood toe to toe with a person in Coffs Harbour a few years ago who was, without doubt, the most evil and abusive person I had ever met. His eyes were full of evil. So there is real evil stuff out there, but depression and mental illness is not demon possession. If it were so, we would have to include biblical champions, people like King David, Elijah, Job, Jonah, and Jeremiah in the category of the demon possessed.

I remember for years, even after becoming a Christ-follower and even as a young preacher, having strong self-destructive thoughts. I would be up on a high place, and these thoughts, clear as crystal, would enter my mind: 'Go on! Just chuck yourself off, you're no good.' It devastated me and the guilt that followed rendered me full of shame. The thoughts would run wild in my mind and I would struggle to hold them in. However, it was no demon, just a large amount of uncontrolled thought life still in the process of being healed.

This is how stupid it gets: I was teaching on this subject in a small country town recently when God showed up and did some amazing things. After spending quite some time with many people after the service, I was heading out the back for a cup of coffee, when a man walked up to me. Now sometimes you can just tell when people are coming up to you with *their* message about your message. What he told me went something like this: "Yeah, depression. Man, I got a CD from (a person who will remain nameless but who is a respected church leader with a large congregation) and he said I needed to visualize the demon of depression in the corner of my room and tell it to be gone in Jesus name."

I will not tell you what I thought, and I certainly didn't say what I thought on that occasion. But where does that stuff come from? I think it is born out of misunderstanding of scripture or a general lack of understanding, plus a 'quick fix mentality' in relation to a long-term issue. Add to that a lack of revelation about who we are in Christ and it becomes the teachings of man rather than of God. These teachings will only cause fear and disappointment, rather than being the truth that sets free.

A few verses before we move on:

Colossians 2:9-10

For in Christ all the fullness of the Deity lives in bodily form, and you have been given fullness in Christ, who is the head over every power and authority.

2 Corinthians 5:17

Therefore, if anyone is in Christ, he is a new creation; the old has gone, the new has come!

Colossians 1:13

For he has rescued us from the dominion of darkness and brought us into the kingdom of the Son he loves.

THE WORD OF GOD IS POWERFUL

A wise older man said to me in the very early days of becoming a Christ follower, "Listen son, you need to read chunks of the Bible." I think this instruction came with, "Get into the New Testament, son." Another wonderful older man gave me my first Bible. He was a member of the Gideon's and he gave me a King James Bible. I appreciated and still do appreciate that gift. The only thing is, being dyslexic, I couldn't read, and the broken reading I could do certainly didn't prepare me for the King James Version of the Bible. It is quite funny to look back into my one-bedroom, converted garage under a house and see the dyslexic young me trying to read all that old English. Thankfully I got my hands on a newer version, and sat for hour after hour reading.

In the early hours of the morning, when my thoughts would run away I would pull out my Bible and start reading, at times the one line over and over again (not on purpose). It was really tough at times. Slowly, by what I believe was a great deal of divine intervention, I became a reasonable reader. It was not instant and still I am not a great reader—just better—as God gave me the ability to do the most important of steps in the renovation of my mind—getting His Word into me.

Isaiah 55:11

So is my word that goes out from my mouth: *It will not return to me empty, but will accomplish what I desire and achieve the purpose for which I sent it.*

The word 'empty' comes from the Hebrew word meaning 'void, in vain or totally without effect'. Therefore God's Word must always have an effect. The choice is always what we do with that effect. If a way is illuminated, it always remains our choice as to whether we walk in the illumination.

Psalm 119:105 (NLT)

Your word is a lamp to guide my feet and a light for my path.

There were many dark times in my early life as a Christ-follower when my mind would try to take me in unhealthy directions. This is when I needed a lamp to guide me, and a light to show me the way.

Being a bit of a movie fan, I love those movies where the hero is lost in the underground sewers, and the only light he has is one lantern held out in front of him as he steps further and further through the blackness. There is potential danger at every corner, and each step could mean great peril. He cannot see far, just another step, but sure enough eventually the tunnel gets lighter and a way out becomes clearer. Although I'm no hero, that describes how I walked many times as a young believer. 'If I can only see where my next step will be,' I thought. 'I want the lantern to be God's Word, so that I know I will be safe. My feet will not stumble and I will not fall if my way is lit by His word.'

Probably the greatest trick the Devil plays on us is to make us think that we can live a successful Christian life without soaking in God's Word. I know, even after being a Christ-follower for over 20 years, that if I stop reading the Scriptures I will weaken very quickly. There is nothing more powerful then the Word of God in our lives.

THE WONDER FOUND IN WEAKNESS

Jesus is all about life, not just existence. We can exist, and perhaps make it through by the skin of our teeth with just church on Sunday, but we will never really live.

John 10:10 (NLT)

The thief's purpose is to steal and kill and destroy. My purpose is to give them a rich and satisfying life.

An abundant life! Jesus shows us how to really live. The Greek denotes that the life described in this passage is far greater than just the act of breathing and existing. When we live by the Word of God we become genuinely alive; full of vigor, strength and life.

Luke 4:4 (KJV)

And Jesus answered him, saying, "It is written, That man shall not live by bread alone, but by every word of God."

We truly begin to live when we realize it's not by bread alone, but by every word that comes from God. When and where Jesus said this is important. This was the first temptation the devil put before Jesus. Jesus' response to this would set up the other temptations. Natural bread will give us strength, but the bread of the Word of God will give us life. Strength and natural bread are no good without spiritual life. Not just air in our lungs, but an abundant and full life.

We live in a download culture. We can get almost anything we want virtually instantly from the internet. How great it would be to just download God's Word into our spirits and find that all problems would be solved. Alas, it does not work quite that way. However, we can use modern technology to help us absorb God's Word. There is so much available if we seek it. Consuming the Word of God is literally hearing God speak. The Bible tells us that '*the Word became flesh*,' John 1:14 so we ascertain by this that Jesus is the living Word.

If we realize that He understands us and our thoughts, and that there is no reason to fear Him, the healing process can take a great step forward. After all, it is God who tells us that there is no condemnation for those who are in Christ Jesus.

I don't know why I persisted in attempting to read God's Word, stuttering and stammering in confusion many times. Not having a television in that little flat did help enormously. All I can say is that God had His hand on me. I do know this; that He heard my cry in the midnight hour and came to equip me to seek Him. The Bible says, '*You said 'seek my face': your face I will seek.*' Psalm 27:8

Psalm 119:10

I seek you with all my heart; do not let me stray from your commands.

Imagine me standing on one side of a great chasm, with God on the other side. The chasm could be dyslexia or depression or a great number of other things. I want to be closer to God but I have a limitation—this chasm—that seems to always cause me to fall short. Should I get upset that God doesn't miraculously jump me over the chasm? Rather, doesn't it make sense that God, whose desire is to walk closer with me, will in fact equip me with the very things I need to build that bridge to cross into greater understanding of God? I have found this to be true: as I draw near to God He in turn draws near to me. We tend to think that God will just zap us to the other side and everything will be okay, when in reality, it's in the learning and the building that the miraculous takes place in our lives.

There are other things that happened in my life and I wonder why I persisted with them. In our church in those days the leader of the service would often say something like, "Let's turn to Ephesians chapter 4, and read around the congregation. We'll start up the back with you, sister, and go down the rows until we finish the chapter." It made me break out in a cold sweat.

I had a friend who said that whenever her church did this, she would get up and run out. Being more spiritual than her, I would stay. (Actually, I was just so in love with Jesus, and thankful for what He did, that if they said that's what you do as a Christ-follower, I said okay.) But I would count the people and add up how many would read a verse before it got to me. Forget learning anything—I was so scared of making a total fool of myself that I'd add up the people, then count down the passage until I found the verse that I was to read, and as quickly as I could, read that one verse as many times as possible while the voices got closer and closer. I always hoped to get '*Jesus wept*', and when I would look at some verse that had those big Bible words like 'propitiation' or 'sanctification', I would panic more. This was a sound method until, sure enough, old brother such-and-such would get so excited that he'd read two or even three verses just before it got to me. Cold sweats, fear and anxiety would grip me and this was in church. Now as a pastor, I don't encourage that practice!

Through all that I am so glad I stayed. I was a full-blown lost soul who was radically converted, fell in love with Jesus, and just wanted to follow Him with everything I had. I didn't know how to 'do religion' or 'do church'. Worship was not hard. I just knew I was messed up and the one who could fix me was Jesus. It's the middle ground, the 'no man's land' that is the most dangerous for a believer. It's the void of a half-existence in God. I truly wonder if this is what the scriptures would refer to as '*a type of godliness, but denying its power*'. 2 Timothy 3:5

Weakness is not wrong if there is a sowing taking place within it. Look at this verse below.

1 Corinthians 15:43

It is sown in dishonor, it is raised in glory; it is sown in weakness, it is raised in power.

Weakness is not an enemy to the purposes of God. It's when we sow God's Word into our lives and weaknesses that God's power will rise in us. He uses the foolish things of this world.

This passage is so encouraging and I have found great comfort in it over the years.

1 Corinthians 1:26-29

Brothers, think of what you were when you were called. Not many of you were wise by human standards; not many were influential; not many were of noble birth. But God chose the foolish things of the world to shame the wise; God chose the weak things of the world to shame the strong. He chose the lowly things of this world and the despised things—and the things that are not—to nullify the things that are, so that no one may boast before him.

If you wrote this verse out as a list, I could tick each thing off one by one. Here again we see that God has chosen the weak and feeble to bring glory to Himself. I think we get it backwards and think that because we are weak and undone, that we are in some way disqualified for the promises and plans of God, when the opposite is closer to the truth. Take a look at the Apostle Paul's understanding:

2 Corinthians 12:7-10

To keep me from becoming conceited because of these surpassingly great revelations, there was given me a thorn in my flesh, a messenger of Satan, to torment me. Three times I pleaded with the Lord to take it away from me. But he said to me, "My grace is sufficient for you, for my power is made perfect in weakness." Therefore I will boast all the more gladly about my weaknesses, so that Christ's power may rest on me. That is why, for Christ's sake, I delight in weaknesses, in insults, in hardships, in persecutions, in difficulties. For when I am weak, then I am strong.

There are all sorts of theories about Paul's thorn in the flesh.

Was it a constant temptation, or a physical weakness like migraine headaches, epilepsy or an eye complaint? The fact is, we don't really know the exact nature of the weakness, but we know what it taught Paul. The things he went through in his body taught him something that is infused throughout Paul's writings, that divine power is best displayed against the backdrop of human weakness. 'Stars shine brighter against the darkest of skies.'

The result is to bring praise and glory to God. This is why problems may not be removed upon our request. God is leading us to a place of understanding that *His* grace is really all we need. Remember how the Bible says this: *'My strength is made perfect in your weakness.'* (2 Corinthians 12:9)

The word weakness is translated as *astheneia*, pronounced as-then -i-ah and meaning 'infirmity, weakness, disease, sickness'. It's interesting that our English word asthma, which is a 'native weakness', is closely related to the Greek definition.

We need to grab this: our physical and mental native weaknesses and frailties are the areas in which God chooses to make known His perfect strength. Our minds, if these are where our native frailties are, become the very places where God chooses to make His greatness shown for all to see His glory!

God is not trying to change the world through the so called 'super-Christian'. He's the God who takes the broken, the messed up, the down trodden, the emotionally unstable, the depressed and the mentally ill and puts a recovery plan in place to bring glory to Himself and amazing change to the person.

When we say to God, "Oh God I'm so messed up," He replies, "Great, I'm brilliant at fixing up." The great renovator wants to reconstruct us to His glory.

It is usually broken people that God uses most. In *Passion and Purity,* Elisabeth Elliot quoted Ruth Stull of Peru:

"If my life is broken when given to Jesus it is because pieces will feed a multitude, while a loaf will satisfy only a little lad."[5]

A BRUISED REED

Isaiah 42:3 (KJV)

A bruised reed shall he not break, and the smoking flax shall he not quench: he shall bring forth judgment unto truth.

Our native weaknesses and frailties, physically, emotionally and mentally, are the areas of miracles through which God chooses to make known his perfect strength.

Matthew 12:20 (NLT)

He will not crush the weakest reedor put out a flickering candle. Finally he will cause justice to be victorious.

Right at the end of the Book of Job in the Old Testament, there is a statement that is incredibly profound in its simplicity. For chapter after chapter we see Job suffering from anguish after anguish, and heartache after heartache, until God speaks. After God has spoken and rebuked him and his so called friends that sat around him in his suffering, Job comes to a conclusion:

Job 42:5

My ears had heard of you but now my eyes have seen you.

The apostle Paul writes:

Ephesians 1:18

I pray that the eyes of your heart may be enlightened, so that you will know what is the hope of His calling, what are the riches of the glory of His inheritance in the saints.

He is bringing us all to a destination where we will see Him

---

5 E Elliot, Passion and Purity, Power Books (Old Tappan, NJ.: Revell, 1984).

more clearly, in and through illness, in a way we would never see Him had we not walked the road. May our minds be open to the truth that out of our weaknesses God can and will bring something wonderful. Healing may not be instant, but rather a process of discovery leading to greater understanding and freedom than we can ever imagine.

THE LONG AND WINDING ROAD

STEP 2: UNDERSTANDING THE PROCESS OF RECOVERY

There are a few ways in which people tend to learn lessons. There is the 'listening to others and learning from them' method; the 'reading about things and learning from what someone has written method' is also popular.

My personal favorite is 'learning it the hard way'! There is another way of describing this particular learning style and that is 'making the silly mistake yourself'. I showed my skill in this particular art when I learned this valuable lesson: a 40 year-old body does not have the same agility as a 16 year-old. The result was a rather painful knee dislocation while playing six-a-side soccer with people half my age. It left me on crutches and needing quite a lengthy recovery time. It happened, it hurt, and my children enjoyed the fact that I had to preach on crutches for a few weeks. To make matters worse, I'm a male, which always means that injuries are far worse, requiring major amounts of attention for the recovery period.

It takes time to recover from injuries just as it takes time to recover from sicknesses. I have a friend whose wife and daughter were in a horrific motor vehicle accident. In just a few moments, through no fault of their own, their world changed as a drunk driver slammed his car into theirs. Miraculously they survived. However, some three years on, they are still in the recovery process. They are in what the Bible calls 'a time to heal'. It's a long process. No one is critical or judgmental about the time or process of their recovery. After all everyone knows these things take time. Why is it then, that when it comes to illness of the mind, we invariably expect people to be instantly cured?

I hope from this chapter, it will become clear that to live a life beyond depression and mental illness will only be possible through a recovery process. In the same way that my knee took a long time to recover, and I could only take small tender steps during the healing process, so we take small tender steps in recovery from depression, mental and emotional illness.

Before we launch into this chapter, let's look at medication for a moment. A very large proportion of people who eventually see a doctor, specialist, or some sort of mental health professional will, in our current environment, be placed on mood-stabilizing medication. In some cases, this medical treatment is necessary and can literally be a lifesaver.

Without doubt, the greatest problem with these types of medication is that some people stop taking them abruptly. This is especially prevalent within some churches, as we hear constantly about the healing power of God. Many feel convicted in their faith and stop their medication quickly. However, to suddenly stop taking mood-stabilizing medication for whatever reason is extremely dangerous. Under no circumstances should anyone who is taking these types of treatments stop taking them instantly. Let me explain. I firmly believe that people who have received faith in Christ should continue to take medication in Jesus' name while recovering. This way, over a period of months or even years, your life will stabilize and grow in Christ to the point that in many cases, the medication can gradually be reduced and hopefully eventually be removed. Medication needs to be seen as a part of the holistic approach to wellness.

The reasoning for not stopping is as follows: everyone has moods, imaginations, ups and downs in life. In this graph we see a regular mind/emotions mix with highs and lows. Obviously the majority of time is spent in the middle area. For want of a better word, let's for the sake of this exercise call this 'normal'.

It might be helpful to describe this visually using the graphs below.

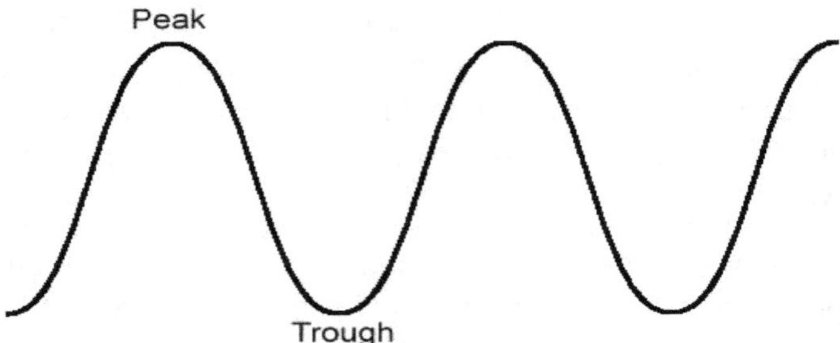

Figure 1: Normal brain/mood function

Many people are either born with, or have, as a result of some trauma, minds that function a little differently. People suffering from bipolar, schizophrenia, depression and the like function more like the graph below. Their peaks are higher and their valleys lower than what we would consider normal.

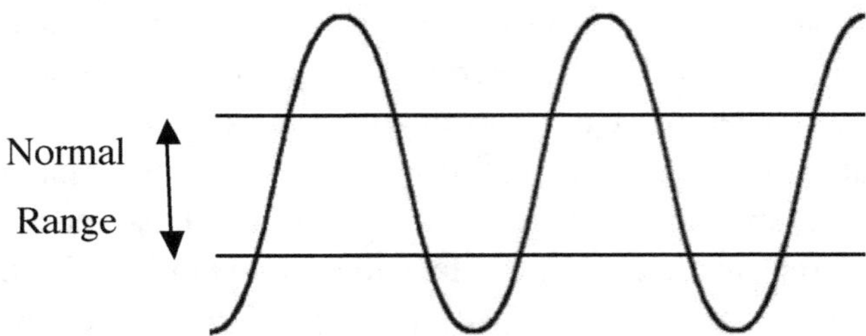

Figure 2: Extreme mood ranges

A mood-stabilizing medication will make the peaks lower and the valleys not as deep. These attempts to stabilize the mind by using medication can be very effective, and in many cases, life saving.

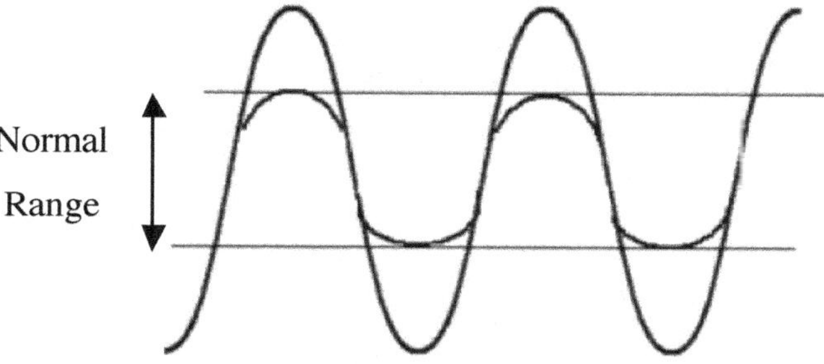

Figure 3: Removal of extreme highs and lows

The danger happens when the medications are removed quickly. Most sufferers will launch into a massive high, almost like the high brought on by a stimulant or an illegal drug. These manic highs and the euphoric feelings they produce can become extremely addictive. When this happens, the sufferer will seem to have enhanced energy and excitement. In this euphoric state they have increased brain activity, as the mind tries to balance out the sudden removal of the artificial chemical administered through medication. There are false feelings of confidence and very often an increased speech rate. I have seen this last for anything from a few hours to days, and sometimes, weeks. It continues until our poor sufferer comes off the peak and very quickly plummets to a low far greater than they experienced before the medication was introduced. At this point, guilt and shame set in. They start to self-destruct and destroy relationships around them. Anger surfaces and they very often shut themselves off from the very people who can help them.

Sadly to say, this is the point at which suicidal thoughts can enter the mind in a more real way. Mix this with self-medicating behavior such as consuming alcohol regularly and in large doses can lead to a very tragic end. These lows are desperate times for so many. All of this can be avoided by remaining on the medication and living with a greater understanding of how healing works in mental and emotional illnesses.

It's true that some of the medications have side effects that are not nice. If your medication reacts with you in ways that cause you anxiety, you should see your doctor as quite often the first medication prescribed may not be the right one for you. We must remember that this is not an exact science. Although we have come a great distance in the understanding of different parts of the brain and its various areas and functions, our understanding is still in its infancy regarding the complexities of thought and emotion.

Of course, it's rare that someone enjoys taking medication. No one likes to take it, especially if they are a believer, and especially if they believe that their mind should be instantly healed with a quick prayer.

Let us dispel the hyper-faith, condemnation-based philosophy that medication is evil. Jesus is known as our great physician after all, and even the disciple Luke was a doctor. I think we should praise God for our medical profession and learn to trust Jesus through the times when we take medical advice.

2 Timothy 1:7 (KJV)

"For God has not given us a spirit of fear; but of power, and of love, and of a sound mind."

Many Bible translations agree that the better translation for 'sound mind' is 'self-discipline'. So we can see a vast difference in how we can understand the scripture as a promise for us, especially if we are a sufferer of a mind that is not 'sound'.

Does God just zap us with a new 'sound mind' upon the receiving of the Holy Spirit at the point of conversion, or is it that the soundness of mind we so desire is actually obtained by 'self-discipline'?

The zapping may seem easier and more desirable, yet self-discipline in the long run is much more beneficial.

If you can grab hold of the principles in this book and implement them into your life, given time, your recovery will be noted by the medical profession. Maybe in the future the medication can be removed, or at least lessened greatly. The reality is that even if you or someone you know has to take medication for the rest of their lives, does it really matter that much? Bearing in mind that our lives are, as the Bible describes in James 4:14, '*but a vapor*', or '*a breath*'. If we go on to live productive, guilt-free, stable lives with good relationships that bring glory to God, does that little bit of medication really matter that much? Very few would feel guilty for taking blood thinning medication, migraine tablets or for that matter, asthma medication. Why should there be such a stigma regarding mood stabilizers? I know that we would all rather not take any medication, however, we should not feel guilty or in any way a lesser person because we take medication to help the healing and recovery process.

I wish I had known this earlier. I remember stirring myself up in faith to believe for healing of my asthma condition, throwing out my medication and, in a very short space of time, ending up in hospital.

UNDERSTANDING RECOVERY IS THE KEY

The word 'recover', according to the Collins dictionary means 'to find again, or obtain the return of something lost'. The word recovery means 'the act or process of recovery, especially from sickness, a shock, or a setback'.

Let us get away from the instant 'blab it and grab it' type of understanding when it comes to things of the emotions and mind. It is a process that will take time and energy, but in the end will make us so much better. I know this could be very hard to see right now, but in the end you will be a better you and a far more useful member of society than ever before. You will also be equipped better for what is needed to fulfill the great mission on earth and be effective for God's kingdom.

BEAUTIFUL IN ITS TIME

Ecclesiastes 3:11

He has made everything beautiful in its time. He has also set eternity in the hearts of men; yet they cannot fathom what God has done from beginning to end.

God is, if we are willing, making us beautiful in our time. Does this mean outward beauty as the world would proclaim it in commercials? When someone realizes the fact that God is creating in them something beautiful, the guilt and shame of suffering from an illness is taken away, and literally their faces lift. The beauty that comes from a heart and mind at peace with God and not living in constant guilt and shame is one of the most beautiful sights on the earth!

In the wedding song of Psalm 45:11 we see this statement: '*The King of kings is enthralled by your beauty.*' We who love God are the bride of Christ, the King of Kings, and believe it or not, when our love is all toward Him, He is enthralled by our beauty. Think about this for a moment: the King of Glory, Jesus, left His beauty (Isaiah 53:2) in order to be able to make us beautiful in our time!

Philippians 2:7-8

...But made himself nothing, taking the very nature of a servant, being made in human likeness. And being found in appearance as a man...

Isaiah 61:3

To bestow on them a crown of beauty instead of ashes, the oil of gladness instead of mourning, and the garment of praise instead of a spirit of despair. They will be called oaks of righteousness, a planting of the LORD for the display of his splendor.

What beautiful imagery we can see here. The word 'beauty' comes from the Hebrew word *peh-ayr,* which relates to a head-dress or bonnet. What a beautiful picture we can see—that God will cover, or even encase our minds in His beauty.

The words 'heaviness', or 'despair', translate as 'darkness, or dim colorless state'. So we can say that when my mind is in darkness, or living in a state of dim colorless existence, God will place a beautiful covering over my mind to display not *my* glory, not *my* beauty, but a beauty far greater—*for the display of his splendor*—to literally bring glory to God.

There is a passage in 1 Peter 3:3-5 that talks about true beauty and yes, this passage does refer to husbands and wives, but we see a key that goes far beyond a marriage only. The fact that God describes us the church as His bride, emphasizes this.

1 Peter 3:3-5 (NLT)

Don't be concerned about the outward beauty of fancy hairstyles, expensive jewelry, or beautiful clothes. You should clothe yourselves instead with the beauty that comes from within, the unfading beauty of a gentle and quiet spirit, which is so precious to God. This is how the holy women of old made themselves beautiful.

In this passage we can see a key to true beauty. I am passionately in love with my wife, Robyn. I love it when she dresses up, puts on some makeup and does her hair. She looks stunning. It's awesome, and I believe that we should always try to look our very best for our partners. But I must say the thing that, when we first met and still today, makes her the most beautiful person in the world is her love and passion for all things Jesus. It is not an 'in your face', 'over the top', extraverted passion. Her nature is, in fact, rather quiet. It's an inner, unfading beauty of a gentle and quiet spirit that draws me to her. Not to say that loud people cannot have that inner beauty as well, it's just that Robyn isn't that way.

UNDERSTANDING SEASONS

In Ecclesiastes 3, we looked at the idea that 'everything is beautiful in its time'. If you look back a few verses in that same chapter of the Bible, you find four wonderful words: 'a time to mend'. If you are suffering from illness, whether it be extreme anxiety attacks, bipolar mood disorder, or low level depression that you may think is just a case of the blues, you are in 'a time to mend.' A time to mend is a good place to be. It's okay!

We need to understand seasons and allow these times to do their work in our lives. It cannot, nor should it, always be spring and summer in our lives. As seasons come and go every year, let us understand that the seasons in our lives are just as real... all four of them. A fool could say, "I don't believe that winter will come," but it will come! Some others may say, "this winter has been so long, I cannot see spring ever arriving." However, spring will come, whether mankind believes it or not! What of those suffering with the bitter cold of depression or mental illness? Take heart, spring will come. To enjoy its warmth and the colors of spring, it will take a stepping from the shadows into the light, but be assured, spring will come. Hold onto that today. It may not come today or tomorrow, but it will come. The snow will melt, the grass will grow, and the flowers will bloom. It's a certainty that as long as this earth we live on keeps turning, then spring times will come. Right back in the beginning of the Bible, God says these words:

Genesis 8:22

While the earth remains, seedtime and harvest, and cold and heat, and summer and winter, day and night, shall not cease.

This is an interesting passage regarding how we should approach seasons in our lives:

Ecclesiastes 11:3-6

If clouds are full of water, they pour rain upon the earth. Whether a tree falls to the south or to the north, in the place where it falls, there will it lie.

Whoever watches the wind will not plant; whoever looks at the clouds will not reap.

As you do not know the path of the wind, or how the body is formed in a mother's womb, so you cannot understand the work of God, the Maker of all things.

Sow your seed in the morning, and at evening let not your hands be idle, for you do not know which will succeed, whether this or that, or whether both will do equally well.

SOWING

We can learn a valuable lesson regarding our approach to depression and mental illness in verse 4. If we spend our time watching the winds and clouds in our lives, we will never plant what needs to be planted; and we will never reap what needs to be reaped.

Now a harvest takes time to grow, just as a recovery takes time to happen. If we break a leg it takes time to recover. Why not let recovery take the time it needs with our minds? For a leg to heal properly it must be set well, and it's the same with our minds; it tends to be how we set our mind while it's healing that makes all the difference. Verse 6 says 'sow your seed in the morning'. These words instruct us, despite the clouds and the winter cold, to sow into our lives seeds that will bring about the right crop in time. Yes, the wind is howling, the rain is falling, the dark clouds are rolling in and times seem terrible right now. But plant what needs to be planted anyway. The harvest, or our recovery, will come in time. I guess that is the essence of this book, that during the recovery, we plant in our lives the seeds of life and wellness that will grow into a recovered life lived beyond the pain of depression and mental illness. Any crop will take time to grow, however it will grow and produce what we need to sustain us in our lives.

If we choose to plant the right things into the soil of our lives today, then it becomes only a matter of time before that right crop grows and is harvested.

We can be fooled by our sight. Look around you. What do you see? We may see the wind and look at the clouds, and let them play a trick on us. If we are constantly making decisions based on situations and circumstances that can change tomorrow, then our life will not plant, and therefore not reap the harvest planned for us. The key is to plant even when all looks bad and not to be so consumed by the wind and the rain that we don't plant the right principles into our lives.

Think about the Apostle Paul's outlook in Corinthians:

2 Corinthians 11:23-27

Are they servants of Christ? (I am out of my mind to talk like this.) I am more. I have worked much harder, been in prison more frequently, been flogged more severely, and been exposed to death again and again. Five times I received from the Jews the 40 lashes minus one. Three times I was beaten with rods, once I was stoned, three times I was shipwrecked, I spent a night and a day in the open sea, I have been constantly on the move. I have been in danger from rivers, in danger from bandits, in danger from my own countrymen, in danger from Gentiles; in danger in the city, in danger in the country, in danger at sea; and in danger from false brothers. I have labored and toiled and have often gone without sleep; I have known hunger and thirst and have often gone without food; I have been cold and naked.

I wonder if in the midst of the sea, bobbing up and down all night, cold and wet with sharks circling around him is when Paul came to an understanding of seasons? (Okay, I added the sharks. We don't know if the sharks were there, but I've watched enough movies to know they're always pretty close!)

In another passage he wrote:

Philippians 4:11-13

I am not saying this because I am in need, for I have learned to be content whatever the circumstances. I know what it is to be in need and I know what it is to have plenty. I have learned the secret of being content in any and every situation, whether well fed or hungry, whether living in plenty or in want. I can do everything through him who gives me strength.

I believe we can sow the right things into our lives even in our darkest times. As Paul spent seasons in prison, I am sure he would have rather been out doing other things. Yet it was during these seasons that he wrote most of his letters that are considered totally—every syllable—inspired by God. So a season in prison for one man changed the world for good for millions of others. It was certainly a case of 'inspiration through incarceration'.

Brother Yun, in his incredible life story, *The Heavenly Man,* describes the events that took him to places very few could bear. He experienced many extremely challenging seasons in his life, yet out of them came a life and story that has changed millions of lives for the better.

Even John Bunyan wrote the classic *Pilgrim's Progress* from a prison cell. I think we see depression and mental illness as a prison cell that we will never be free from. That is not a correct understanding. Out of the cell of the mind can come the most amazing tales of grace, love and redemption that will change the world.

There is an old saying that I heard many years ago and has stuck with me: 'Two men looked through prison bars, one saw mud, the other stars.' What was the difference? Simply the way they were looking. It's the direction of their focus. They were in the same situation yet chose to look in very different directions.

Ecclesiastes 7:14 (NASB)

In the day of prosperity be happy, but in the day of adversity consider-God has made the one as well as the other so that man will not discover anything that will be after him.

Ecclesiastes 7:14 (MSG)

On a good day enjoy yourself; on a bad day, examine your conscience. God arranges for both kinds of days so that we won't take anything for granted.

These verses talk of seasons in our lives and the fact that God is intertwined within them.

THE NEED TO SEE SOVEREIGNTY IN SEASONS

There is a young woman by the name of Esther in the Bible who became a very courageous queen. I encourage you to read her whole story. Perhaps you're just like her and born for 'such a time as this'. The Bible tells us that Esther was taken to undergo beauty treatments that lasted a year before she was even presented before the king. What if, in our lives, the difficulty of depression or mental illness is a 'beauty treatment' that may last years, so that when we come before the King of glory, our beauty, or mainly His beauty within us, is made ready for 'such a time' as God has planned?

Remember the truth of this; 'He has made everything beautiful in its time.'

Working in and through depression and mental illness, I look back now and see that it took a long time for God to mend or 'beautify' this very broken person. While going through the process, I did not think that what I'm about to say would ever be possible. But now I see that all that time God was working, changing, growing, fixing, repairing and renovating to make it possible for someone such as me, the most messed up person on planet earth, to be in the right place at the right time 'for such a time as this', and to show the splendor of God's glory. I don't pretend to fully understand it all. But from beyond it, I can see God in it!

GOD IN THE FIERY FURNACE

Those famous men of faith, Shadrach, Meshach and Abednego, were thrown into a fiery furnace by King Nebuchadnezzar. But there was another (God himself), with them in the heat of this trial. Notice how King Nebuchadnezzar saw God clearly from outside the furnace.

Daniel 3:24-2

Then King Nebuchadnezzar leaped to his feet in amazement and asked his advisers, "Weren't there three men that we tied up and threw into the fire?" They replied, "Certainly, O king." He said, "Look! I see four men walking around in the fire, unbound and unharmed, and the fourth looks like a son of the gods."

I can see now, from beyond the heat, that in my fiery furnace, one like the Son of God walked with me. Even this book has taken over 20 years of healing and recovery to be able to be written. I don't know why it took so long. I suspect that I am a very slow learner (my way of saying I'm a bit thick) and hopefully your journey will be shorter. There is so much I don't understand, but I know that the seasons have changed. In C S Lewis' classic book, *The Lion, the Witch and the Wardrobe,* it talks of a time in the land of Narnia where it is always winter, but never Christmas. Your winter may still be cold and it may have gone on for year after year. But I wish to encourage you today with the knowledge that, if you want them to, the seasons are changing. The wintery fog is lifting. Even the fact that you are reading this book is a step closer to spring, and eventually Christmas will come.

Now in these seasons, or let's call them 'times of recovery', there are certain principles we need to follow to reach the land of clearer skies beyond the rolling banks of fog—a land beyond depression and mental illness.

Someone once said: "If we always do what we've always done, we will always get what we've always got."

Another wise person described the definition of insanity as: "To do the same thing over and over and expect a different result."

I have a history of chronic chest infections. So imagine this: I've been out playing soccer in the rain and I catch a chill and a subsequent cold. I go to the doctor and he or she says, "Now listen, Gary. You need to be careful. You know your history of chest infections and pneumonia." Then the doctor proceeds to give me instructions to keep warm, stay out of the cold night air and take my antibiotic medication three times a day for the full course of the medication. "Yes, yes, yes!" I say, thinking I know better. "I'll be okay." So I decide to go out in sub-zero temperatures and sleeting rain in a thin T-shirt and shorts and only take the medication until I feel a bit better. What do you think might happen to me? Yes, you guessed it—a chest infection, pneumonia and possibly premature death. (A bit morbid I know, but I want to make a point).

Let us not take this approach to our mental wellness recovery

plan. For some of us it took over 20 years to mess our minds up, so how ridiculous is it to think that with a prayer and a bottle of medication that everything will be fine.

Here is a fascinating passage relating to a long term sickness; the healing at the pool of Bethesda:

John 5:1-14 (MSG)

Soon another Feast came around and Jesus was back in Jerusalem. Near the Sheep Gate in Jerusalem there was a pool, in Hebrew called Bethesda, with five alcoves. Hundreds of sick people—blind, crippled, paralyzed—were in these alcoves. One man had been an invalid there for thirty-eight years. When Jesus saw him stretched out by the pool and knew how long he had been there, he said, "Do you want to get well?"

The sick man said, "Sir, when the water is stirred, I don't have anybody to put me in the pool. By the time I get there, somebody else is already in."

Jesus said, "Get up, take your bedroll, start walking." The man was healed on the spot. He picked up his bedroll and walked off.

That day happened to be the Sabbath. The Jews stopped the healed man and said, "It's the Sabbath. You can't carry your bedroll around. It's against the rules."

But he told them, "The man who made me well told me to. He said, 'Take your bedroll and start walking."

They asked, "Who gave you the order to take it up and start walking?" But the healed man didn't know, for Jesus had slipped away into the crowd.

A little later Jesus found him in the Temple and said, "You look wonderful! You're well! Don't return to a sinning life or something worse might happen."

After the healing, Jesus found the man again and instructed him to make a life change. This is because if a change in behavior does not follow healing, we put ourselves in harm's way again. It's like a smoker who receives a miraculous healing from lung cancer yet returns to the habit again, or an alcoholic who is set free from alcohol only to keep going to pubs and clubs.

Through the next chapters there are a series of practical steps to take in the recovery process.

PATIENCE

One of the principles we need to grab hold of is that the promises of God are not obtained by faith alone. The question is asked, 'how do we inherit the promises of God?' The answer, according to the scripture, is through these two things: faith and patience.

Hebrews 6:12 (NLT)

Then you will not become spiritually dull and indifferent. Instead, you will follow the example of those who are going to inherit God's promises because of their faith and endurance.

No one likes the patience part. We are probably all a bit like the guy who knelt beside his bed and prayed, "Dear God, give me patience. And I want it now." God is creating something beautiful in you and even if you don't see it now, that's okay.

If this is your journey, then be patient. Stir your faith and be patient in God. Know that the dark days will still happen, the pain will still surface from time to time and feelings of despair will try to overwhelm you. But stay the course and be patient, planting what needs planting, and we will see the miraculous hand of God bring you through.

One of my all time favorite quotes is from a man known as the prince of preachers, Mr. Charles Haddon Spurgeon. He suffered from depression and anxiety attacks for a very long time. These were so severe that many times he could not get out of his bed. Yet while living with constant mental health challenges, he was able to influence the world greatly for good. He said this:

"God is too good to be unkind. He is too wise to be confused. If I cannot trace His hand, I can always trust His heart."

Do you have a favorite place to eat? I do. It is not fancy, nor expensive. It's in a little county town called Goulburn, about two hours drive from Sydney, Australia, and it's called the Paragon Restaurant. This family-owned restaurant serves lots of great meals, but my favorite is the pepper steak. Without doubt, it is *the* greatest pepper steak I have ever eaten. Normally I like being a bit of a habit breaker. I'll drive a different way to get places and stop at different rest stops. But when it comes to this place, I don't even look at the menu any more. It's what I order. Even now I'm getting hungry for one and I'm about 500 miles away. It's one of those meals that send the taste buds into rapturous delight. Every mouthful is touched with the dew of heaven itself. I can almost hear the *Hallelujah Chorus* rising as angels descend with knife and fork in hand.

Now consider this; God's design is not to turn you into a burger that's slapped together, has very little nutritional value and is consumed quickly. God's design for us, whether we realize it or not, is to make us beautiful in His time. You're a Paragon pepper steak in preparation, and that's a very good thing.

GOD'S HEART IS FOR YOU!

First and foremost God's heart is for you. I was talking to a friend and fellow minister the other day, and he made a statement regarding the names in the Bible. The genealogies are lists of names that we come across in the Bible. If you're like me, you tend to skip over them rather quickly. Even pronouncing most of these names is difficult. God gave this friend a revelation and he said something to the effect of, "Just look at the names—God is all about names, otherwise why are they listed? These were individuals, and God is all about the individual." He knows your name, He knows the hairs on your head and even if your follicles have been in recession like mine, He still knows how many there are.

In Proverbs 18:24, God is described as '*one who sticks closer than a brother.*' In Psalm 139 there are many great statements regarding the understanding of God, and how closely He is entwined within us. Look at some of the wording used to describe the closeness of God to us:

Psalm 139: 1-5

You have searched me and you know me, you know when I sit and when I rise, you perceive my thoughts. You discern and are familiar with all my ways. My words you know completely before I speak them. You hem me in-behind and before, you have laid your hand upon me.

This entire Psalm means so much to me. I will share sections that personally have imparted life to me over the years while traveling through some very dark places.

Verses 11 and 12

If I say, "Surely the darkness will hide me and the light become night around me, even the darkness will not be dark to you; and night will shine like the day, for darkness is as light to you."

I cannot tell you in words what those verses have meant to me in my darkest times. Even typing this, I know it is an insufficient attempt to bring to life something that I will be eternally grateful for, and cannot even with all the eloquence of the written words, ever adequately express. It really is amazing to know that God is with you in the darkest of places. The only problem with that is that it generally means you have had to go through some pretty dark places to realize He's there!

Eight words at the end of verse 18 also contain volumes for me personally: 'When I awake, I am still with you.' My life was constantly filled with the fear of being alone. To know and understand that the God of all creation sits with me even while I sleep and that '*he never sleeps or slumbers*' but is always with me is something that has had a profound effect in my personal life. To know that when my eyes open, God is still with me, is one of the most beautiful and graphic illustrations of God's heart for my life.

GOD LOVES GOOD COFFEE

If you are a true coffee lover, not only are you so much more godly than others, but you will know that the words 'instant' and 'coffee' should never be connected! Isn't 'instant coffee' an oxymoron anyway? True lovers of coffee will spend the time. They will grind the beans, delicately preparing the machine, and while brewing the coffee they will float around in a state of rapturous expectation, breathing in the pure fragrance of the 'nectar of the gods'. (Either that, or they will be anxiously pacing the floor shaking, while sweating on their next caffeine fix.) It takes time to do it right, and guess what? So do you!

You are a work in progress and God is faithful to you. He is perhaps grinding or preparing, but all the time He's in the process of brewing the perfect you.

Being convinced that God is for us and working for our good is a major step forward for all who suffer with depression and mental illness. This is because our minds will try to trick us into thinking that God does not care or is not interested in our issues or sicknesses. This could not be further from the truth. Think about the thing that Jesus did more than anything else as He ministered; He healed sickness. In fact, at one point He made this statement: 'It's not the healthy that need a doctor but the sick.' He goes on to say that He came for the sick. The sick of our world are the closest ones to the heart of God. Let us be convinced of God's heart being toward us.

2 Timothy 1:12

That is why I am suffering as I am. Yet I am not ashamed, because I know whom I have believed, and am convinced that he is able to guard what I have entrusted to him for that day.

TAKING STEPS TOWARD HEALING

This passage tells an amazing little story that we must grab a point from before moving on:

Luke 17:11-19 (MSG)

It happened that as he made his way toward Jerusalem, he crossed over the border between Samaria and Galilee. As he entered a village, ten men, all lepers, met him. They kept their distance but raised their voices, calling out, "Jesus, Master, have mercy on us!"

Taking a good look at them, he said, "Go, show yourselves to the priests." They went, and while still on their way, became clean. One of them, when he realized that he was healed, turned around and came back, shouting his gratitude, glorifying God. He kneeled at Jesus' feet, so grateful. He couldn't thank him enough—and he was a Samaritan.

Jesus said, "Were not ten healed? Where are the nine? Can none be found to come back and give glory to God except this outsider?" Then he said to him, "Get up. On your way. Your faith has healed and saved you."

There are lots of great things we can read into this passage, with some beautiful lessons on gratitude and calling in time of need. However I would like us to consider these points. Firstly, these men were not instantly healed. Could Jesus have instantly healed them? Absolutely. Then there must be a reason why he didn't. Just look what Jesus asked them to do. He asked them to show themselves to the priests, the very thing you would do if you were cleansed. The reason for this was so the priest could ratify that you were able to return to your family and life in general. The only thing is, they had not been healed yet. Or had they? Jesus had spoken into their lives already. Jesus instructed them to do something that would only be done by a healed person. He wanted to see if they would act on his instructions without the visible signs of change in their bodies.

We also need to act on His instructions, even if we don't see instantly the healing He has promised. It was in the obedience to what Jesus said that their healing came. As a parallel, it is in the obedience to the principles laid out here in this book that are backed by scripture, which is God-breathed, that the healing will come in and on the journey. This is the key in recovery: acting upon God's instructions even before seeing an outward change.

I like to imagine those men walking away from Jesus still covered with leprosy. The doubts and fears must have risen as they must have walked quite a distance before realizing they were clean. We can see this, because nine of the men didn't bother to return to thank Jesus. If it were only up the road they would all have run back to thank Him.

Jesus had told them to do something before they could see the healing. This Jesus, whom they had heard of, as well as all the testimonies that filtered through to them of his great miracles, had told them to do something that only a healed person should do. Yet, he had not instantly cleansed them. Why? We can only speculate on what they thought, but they were human and subject to all the fears and doubts we have. It's like understanding seasons. The leprosy is still there, but we can choose to obey His voice and start walking anyway. We start walking and start planting into our lives as we travel along this road to recovery, even while we are still ill—taking the right steps, even though nothing seems different yet.

THE GREATER GOOD

The healing of the ten lepers is a very important miracle and is known as a 'Messianic' miracle. For over 1,500 years, there had been a protocol in place to pronounce a person clean who had an infectious skin disease. You can find all the details in Leviticus chapter 14. It was an amazing process. These ten men would have sparked a full investigation with animal sacrifices, bodily shavings, proclamations and all sorts of rituals. Now think about this: Jesus could have healed them instantly, and that would have been good. However, in the delay of the healing, and the process of walking in obedience to God's instructions, far more people witnessed the miraculous, and the effect confirmed that Jesus is the Messiah.

I believe that God is proving His greatness and proclaiming His glory through the process of recovery as we walk in his instructions.

GOD'S DELAYS ARE NOT GOD'S DENIALS

What if the delay of your healing means that the goodness of God is proclaimed to a nation, rather than just an individual? Healing will come, as sure as day follows night.

These men had a choice—do I do what Jesus instructs me to do, even though I don't see my healing right now? They could have shrugged their shoulders and gone off in a huff just because they were not instantly healed. They could have been thinking, 'That didn't work. So much for Jesus! I will die in my leprosy'. But they would have been profoundly wrong, as healing was theirs as they walked in God's instructions.

LOOK AT IT AS FOR A SEASON

Grab this hope, and let this be the first planting along this pathway to recovery, that there is hope for a life beyond depression and mental illness. It takes time and seasons, yet I know there is such a place. Not because someone said so, or because I read it in a book. I live there now and it's a beautiful place.

These steps we have come to see together:

- Understanding that life beyond depression and mental illness is not obtained by a quick fix.
- There is a road to recovery before each of us and we must begin to walk that road, even if what we see outwardly has not yet changed.
- Planting into our lives the seed that, given time and seasons, will produce a good crop.
- If we choose to plant the right things into the soil of our lives today, then it becomes only a matter of time before that right crop grows and is harvested.

COOL RUNNINGS

STEP 3: ANSWERING THE VALUE QUESTION

The value of a person is not dependant on the sum of their accomplishments.

I have puzzled as to why, in our modern western culture, we have over recent years developed such alarming rates of depression, mental illness and emotional instability. There has always been depression and mental illness in our human nature. Yet why such an alarming increase over recent years? Why does this coincide with a period of prolonged prosperity in our nation and most of the western or developed societies? We now take for granted as normal things that only a few decades ago would have been considered luxurious and perhaps out of reach for many 'normal' folk.

Yet in the midst of all this prosperity, we have witnessed the destruction of the family unit. Where a child at school with only one parent used to be a rarity, now, one who has both their natural parents living under the same roof as a family unit has become the rarity. Marriage breakdown is prolific, and the number of people suffering from mental-related illness has soared, making depression and mental illness probably our greatest health concern.

According to the World Health Organization, mental illness is the number one health concern facing our society. A recent report[5] quoted the Mental Health Council of Australia as saying, "Medicare figures show an alarming 40 percent increase in the number of Medicare claims for mental health consultations since the global financial crisis started". This in a nation that has, in large, averted the worst of the devastating effects shown in other western nations.

Certainly in part, the reason we have seen such an alarming rate of increase in mental-related illness, marriage and family unit breakdown and escalating numbers of suicides and all forms of violence including domestic, road rage and homicide, is that somewhere in the world of prosperity and wealth we have come to believe that our value as human beings is based on the sum of our achievements and accomplishments. It is no wonder we have believed this lie. Constantly we are bombarded with images of the successful and desirable. Advertising and television consistently feed this misconception. The perfect skin, the newest car, the greatest body, the perfect partner, etcetera. These are not necessarily bad things, in and of themselves, however if we take our personal value from these things, it's no wonder we always come up short.

Our value somehow became based on our looks, our partner and their looks, and the things we own. This is why we have a world full of people living in poor relationships and giving their bodies away, because they actually believe that they are not worth anything without that relationship. We see people selling out their ethics for the sake of financial gain and others destroying their homes and families through gambling and wasteful living.

---

5 Mental illness soars as global crisis hits By Jennifer Macey for "AM" Posted Mon May 4

SEX

Our TVs preach at our youth that pre-marital sex is okay and in fact should be done. It says that you can run from relationship to relationship and give your body away without it affecting your spirit or soul. "It's just sex," they will say. The truth is that sex is anything but 'just sex'. Sex is a wonderful thing and I'm a huge fan. To have a great sexual relationship within the beauty of a holy marriage is, I think, the closest thing to heaven on earth. Sex is not 'just sex' and the messages preached by our TVs are so destructive that we see lives wasted every day because of this messed-up understanding. We have thousands of amazing young people who see their personal value as only as good as the girlfriend or boyfriend they have, and that they are in some way a loser if they don't have one.

BODY IMAGE

Body image is another area of concern and misleading information. Today in our society, if a young woman is of a more solid build, she can suffer from all sorts of negative feelings toward herself because she doesn't have the doctored, fake, breast-implanted, supposedly perfect figure. Who said that the image we see in the magazines and on TV is the 'perfect' figure anyway? The end result of all this incorrect propaganda has led a generation into all sorts of eating disorders, depression and suicide because they can't live up to the perceived level of expectation within society.

THE SUCCESS MENTALITY

The success mentality within our modern culture is a major concern. Success is a great thing, and should always be encouraged. However, when society reaches a point where we have business people destroying their families for the sake of earning extra money, working crazy hours to drive the right car and have the right stuff, all this becomes counter productive to the real meaning of life and happiness.

Now don't get me wrong here. I am an adamant believer in success. It is a great thing to achieve in the business world, and some people are incredibly gifted in that area. More power to them. The problem is not in the success, but rather if we see our value as dependent upon the success. If our value as a person is based on the success we achieve, then we start messed-up already. We start from the wrong foundation and a faulty foundation. To use a building example, we can build the greatest and most glamorous sky scraper ever constructed, but if the foundations are flawed, even the greatest of manmade projects with the most picturesque facades will come tumbling down. The Bible warns us about what it calls 'putting trust in wealth that can vanish.' 1 Timothy 6:17

I must confess I believed this lie also. I fell for it with everything I had. In fact I became a passionate preacher of this philosophy. Wealth and success were tied together and unable to be separated in my understanding. These were the way to happiness and the secret to a fulfilled life. If I became wealthy enough, everything would be fine. I'd have that happiness I'd always wanted. Life was all about image and wealth, having the right car, the right girl and the right stuff. I remember (and so do my parents unfortunately) the day I told my Mum and Dad that because they were over 40 and not millionaires, they had failed in life. We laugh about it now, but I believed it and stood them up in the kitchen and let them have it. I believed the lie; I believed it with every fiber of my being. When you believe that it's all about wealth and success and it falls apart, what do you do?

My passion is that by the end of this chapter, you will have a greater and clearer understanding of your value. Not a false outward appearance-based value, but rather a genuine understanding of your value simply for who you are.

One of the greatest days in my life was the day I realized that my value is not in what others think. It's not in the car I drive or the house I own. It's certainly not in my waist line or my hair. My waist line I'm working on, but the hair's gone! Please take time to really consider this. Our value, our *true* value is found in the love of our God for us, just simply because of who we are.

I appreciate success and promote it. I have spoken at conferences and trained people in the art of success. *Get Out There,* use *The Power of Positive Thinking*, and *The Magic of Thinking Big*. I want to *See You at the Top,* and even *Over the Top. High Five*-ing, *Influencing People* and even *Becoming a Rain Maker* while you're at it, and if you can *Retire Young and Retire Rich* and get the *Cash Flow Quadrant* all *Revved* up, go for it! (The words in italics are successful book titles). However, it is an empty thing if we trust these things for our value as a person.

Please, be as successful as you can. If your gift is business, then use that gift for all its worth, as it truly is a gift. Use it to bring strength and security to as many as you can. The great John Wesley once wrote:

'Do all the good you can, by all the means you can, in all the ways you can, in all the places you can, at all the times you can, to all the people you can, as long as ever you can.'

I'm an adamant believer in success and financial growth. It's the context and the priorities that are my concern.

Let me explain it this way. The movie *Cool Runnings* is a classic comedy based on a true story. Hopefully you have seen this movie, if not, stop everything and see it!

It's based on the incredible story of the Jamaican bobsled team going to the winter Olympics. The team's coach who in years gone by was a great bobsled driver, had been disgraced after having had his gold medals taken off him for cheating. The night before the gold medal run, young Doreas, the driver of the bobsled team, asked the coach why he cheated. The coach, after describing how he had made winning his whole life, and how he had to win at all costs no matter what, makes this statement: "A gold medal is a wonderful thing. But if you're not enough without it, you'll never be enough with it."

Success and achievement is like that. It's a wonderful thing! But if we are not enough without it, we will never be enough with it. If our value is based in our accomplishments or our wealth, then what happens if our wealth vanishes and our accomplishments fail? Why do many who have achieved great things still fall into depression and mental illness? Why do seemingly successful people live in a state of despair year after year? As good as it is to aspire to and achieve bigger, better and brighter things, like that gold medal, 'if you're not enough without it, you'll never be enough with it'.

Our value simply as a person is of a higher value than all the gold this world can offer. You are enough, by just being. The Bible gives us some incredible pictures of our true value. Let's look at the biblical illustration of the lost coin:

Luke 15:8-10

Or suppose a woman has ten silver coins and loses one. Does she not light a lamp, sweep the house and search carefully until she finds it? And when she finds it, she calls her friends and neighbors together and says, 'Rejoice with me; I have found my lost coin.' In the same way, I tell you, there is rejoicing in the presence of the angels of God over one sinner who repents.

The coin's value was not in its situation. It was a valued coin, whether in the woman's hand, around her neck, or on the floor in some forgotten corner of the house. Its value as a coin was in the value of itself as a coin, created and stamped with its value by the coin's creator.

The coin is stamped with the image of the king and that image defines the value of the coin. As with all of us, it's the image of a king—the King of Kings—imprinted on every fiber of our DNA that shows our value.

We are all coins created to be of value. We may find throughout life that we have ended up lost, covered in dirt, messed up and not where we think we should be. This may be true, but we are still valuable coins. We are stamped with a value by the Creator.

Although the coin was lost, the value of the coin was never lost. The built-in fundamental value of the coin was not dependent upon the circumstances the coin found itself in. God wants us to realize this. He describes how this lady lights a lamp so she can see into even the dark places. She sweeps the house using energy and effort. She searches carefully until she finds it. She does not stop until this coin is found. Even in the search, we see the value placed on us.

If we go back a few verses we see the story of the lost sheep:

Luke 15:3-7 (NLT)

So Jesus told them this story: "If a man has a hundred sheep and one of them gets lost, what will he do? Won't he leave the ninety-nine others in the wilderness and go to search for the one that is lost until he finds it? And when he has found it, he will joyfully carry it home on his shoulders. When he arrives, he will call together his friends and neighbors, saying, 'Rejoice with me because I have found my lost sheep.' In the same way, there is more joy in heaven over one lost sinner who repents and returns to God than over ninety-nine others who are righteous and haven't strayed away!

Can you see the heart of God in these passages and, more than that, the value of every single person on this earth, no matter what their circumstances? What distance has God traveled, or is still traveling, to find *you,* simply because you are of such value to Him? The fact that Jesus left heaven and crossed the cosmos to rescue us is astounding. Others may not value us, but God does and that is what really matters.

If who I am and my value is based on other people's opinions and expectations, then I will never be able to live up to that. I will always see myself as less than able. This is why we must see our value from God's view point. This is what really matters, and this understanding will shape our lives and change our mindsets better than anything else. I know that sounds simplistic, however it's true nonetheless! I personally struggled with this for a long time.

In our western culture these stories may have played out more like this: "Oh, I have nine other coins. I'll deposit them and earn some interest, and before long that lost coin will be replaced. It's all okay." Or, "I still have 99 sheep and they'll breed soon. I will be getting some more, so that stupid rebellious sheep? I'll just forget about it and leave it. I'll have more than 100 soon anyway."

This is how *we* might think, and that methodology may have sound business sense within it. But this is not how God works. He values each and every one, and it's His will that none should remain lost. How amazing it is that God never writes us off?

Let's get really real about this. Do you see yourself as enough?

Can you honestly look in the mirror and say you actually like yourself, warts and all? (Actually no one really likes warts, but I think you know what I mean). Let's be real. This took me a long time, even as a passionate Christ-follower, to understand. You can probably tell if you think you're enough by that voice in the back of your head that's telling you to shut the book right now. No, don't do it! Keep reading! This will change your life in a more positive way than anything else ever can.

Our value is far more than our wealth, our accomplishments or our toys (I threw that in for us men). Come on, let's get real. If we can just see this more clearly, we will take a huge step forward. The fact that Christ placed a value so high on each of us as individuals, that He would leave heaven with all its greatness, wealth, majesty and grandeur to come to this earth with the express mission of dying the most agonizing and horrific of deaths, to show us the value God places on us, still amazes me.

Around the time I became a Christ-follower there was a song around that went something like this; 'He could have called ten thousand angels to destroy the world and set Himself free. He could have called ten thousand angels, but He died alone for you and for me.'

We can judge our effectiveness in our various fields of expertise by our accomplishments, and so we should. To judge our personal value in the same way is foolishness.

I have often said, taught, and lived with the understanding that generally the higher you go up in an organization, the better the people are. This is generally true if we are judging the quality by given mindsets, mentalities and attitudes. But it is fundamentally flawed to see the value of a person in this light.

The value of an individual person, whether a billionaire CEO of a multinational corporation, or a young single mum from a broken home living in government housing, with three children to different fathers, is the same. We are valued simply because we are, each of us knitted together in our mother's womb.

Let's discuss failure for a moment.

There are very few things in this world I do well, however, on this subject I would consider myself well-qualified. In fact over the years, failure has been a bit of a specialty of mine. It's a gift, what can I say!

Consider this story:

Someone approaches the city gate.

"Who goes there, friend or foe?" comes the cry from the watchman. The reply comes swiftly, "What would you have me be, for I can be either."

"Explain yourself, sir, for you are armed as prepared for battle yet your sword is not drawn."

The reply comes, "To some I am a friend, to some a bitter enemy. Do you not know me, for I dwell in this city, for I have always been with you? In great triumph I have fought beside you, yet at other times I have caused you to cower and hide. All great men know me and have learnt from me and mastered me, yet others have let me be their master and yes, I am a cruel master. Now wise gate keeper, how will you take me? Am I your friend or your foe?"

"Tell me your name sir, for how can I recognize you unless your name be given?"

"My name is failure."

From the moment I became a Christ-follower, I knew I would preach God's word. As strange as it is that God would choose a dyslexic, insecure, mentally unstable, broken and totally messed-up person, I just knew. So coming from the state I was in, I launched into telling everyone how amazing God is. I would walk the streets of Coffs Harbour at night, telling anyone I could about how God had changed me. I went to the pastor of the church and asked if I could preach. He said okay and I got ready. I preached for about 15 minutes, and everyone praised my zeal and passion for Christ. Now I know there are some pastors reading this and the red lights are flashing right about now, and *you* may be thinking, 'Oh no!' Well, precisely. This great moment went straight to my head. It is amazing how quickly things change from being a humble, thankful, willing, grace-filled, compassionate young man to 'I'm God's gift to the pulpit'. As you can imagine my next effort was rather less well-received and finished with utter humiliation and embarrassment. It was one of those 'wishing the ground would open up and swallow me' moments. I told you, it's just a gift of mine. I had messed up royally and had to live with these people who now realized what a big bag of wind I really was. I had failed, and certainly would have to wait a long time before they let this boy behind the pulpit again. Although I felt that I was a failure, I was not. True, I had failed, but failure is an event, never a person.

Abraham Lincoln once wrote:

'My great concern is not that you have failed, but whether you are content with your failures.'

These quotes have given me great comfort many times:

'A flawed diamond is always more valuable than a perfect house brick.'

'Failure is an event, not a person.'

This step of understanding our true value is vital on the road to recovery and a life beyond mental, emotional and depressive-related illnesses. So much of depression and mood disorders are founded in our lack of self worth. If the expectation of God was perfection, He would never have rescued me!

Be it the high end of achievement or the low end, it's still the same. If we judge our value in terms of success and/or failure in business or personal life, then when a business goes well we are of value, but what about when a marriage fails? What do we do when our mistakes and regrets come tumbling down on us as we lie awake in worry and sadness? This is when the understanding of our true value will anchor our lives through turbulent circumstances. I guess what really made me realize this was an incident regarding one of our daughters.

OUR LITTLE GIRL

About a year after Robyn and I married, we moved from Coffs Harbour, to the beautiful city of Ballarat in Victoria. We started our family at roughly the same time I started a business in carpet cleaning. We were functioning in the voluntary role of youth pastors in a local small church as well. Our eldest daughter Laura arrived, followed by Sarah a little less than two years later, followed then by Rachel another two years on. Things were going well. The youth group was growing, we were busy, and our three little girls were awesome.

One night a curve ball hit our family in the shape of one of our girls having her first grand mal epileptic seizure. This was the beginning of what proved to be many years of battling this very confusing and heartbreaking illness. We don't know what sparked it, but all of a sudden we were walking a road that was truly heart breaking. The questions raged in my mind. Was it the trauma of losing my younger brother to cancer while she was in the womb? Did that stressful time contribute? Was it a fall or something we did or didn't do as parents? At first we thought it was perhaps a sickness-related side effect, or did someone leave some medication around that she swallowed? Without going through all the details, this was the start of many years dealing with a child having epilepsy.

None of this—the pediatricians, blood tests, other tests and scans, the medication that, at times, would so suppress her mind that education was very difficult due to constant sleepiness—none of this fit into my theology as a preacher and a young stirred up Christ-follower. If I lay hands on the sick they will recover, or so my Bible tells me. During this time we would have amazing things happen. I remember in a church service that I was leading once, my amazing, life-filled young girl went into a seizure sitting in the front row. We prayed for her, the seizure stopped instantly and supernaturally and instead of her falling asleep for hours after the seizure, (which was the normal pattern), she was wide awake and excited, as if nothing had happened. Was this a healing or a partial healing? At other times we would pray and the seizures would not stop, and even seem to get worse.

During a particular period, her seizures became increasingly worse and more frequent. The doctors raised her medication again and were troubled by what was happening. We were very worried. We would pray and hope for the best. The intensity seemed to be increasing sharply, and our pediatrician was very concerned. I don't know when the word tumor was mentioned, however the signs were not promising. I don't know why, but I thought there was a distinct possibility that we might be losing her. I remember kneeling beside my bed and praying a prayer that no parent should ever have to pray. "Lord, if this is her time to go, please take her quickly so she will not suffer anymore."

We were booked into a clinic in Liverpool, Western Sydney, for another test. This one would reveal if there was a tumor in her brain. So we asked a select group who we knew really would pray for her, to pray. We didn't go telling everyone; sometimes it simply hurt too much to do that.

The day came, these people were praying for our beautiful girl and something happened that day. I cannot explain it. They found a place where there may have been something, a slight scarring at the back of her brain and from that day, the seizures stopped! It was nothing short of a miracle, as there was no other way to explain what happened. For a few years, from that day, she didn't have another epileptic fit; her medication was reduced and eventually stopped all together. The change was so dramatic that after a period of time we wrote letters to people proclaiming how amazing and miraculous her healing was.

But, when this beautiful young lady hit puberty, our nemesis returned. Now this does not fit in any theological textbooks. An undeniable miracle followed by more sickness. I don't have an answer for you. Sorry. It's just the way things unfolded. I think we all like to pin point blame and fault, and establish cause and effect. I simply don't know why, but I do know now, that God can use the most hurtful things we go through, to bring about the miraculous.

One such occasion, though utterly heartbreaking, became a moment in my life that I still, many years later, remember vividly. This moment became what I consider the point where I realized the value God places on me, and in turn, each of us.

I was preparing to leave on a work trip from Campbelltown in Sydney's south west, to Cowra (about four hours away) to speak. I was going to leave early Thursday morning, and the subject I was speaking on was divine healing. Our daughter was quite sick during this time and I know that Robyn and I spent many years half-sleeping, as she would have seizures in her sleep. It was the Wednesday evening before I was to leave, and our little girl, now about seven years old, had a long and difficult seizure. I'm talking scarily long. It just wouldn't stop. Words cannot describe the utter helplessness a parent feels in that situation.

After what seemed such a long time, (and they all seemed long but this one was nasty) I picked up her now totally limp body, and carried her from her room. As I walked through the house I just wept, shattered again by this sickness. I just wanted it to stop. This thorn was just too hard and it hurt too much. The next day, those hours in the car passed extremely slow, as a broken father questioned His God, got angry, cried, thought, tried to figure this out and just plain hurt. I didn't realize that I was about to learn a lesson from God through this illness that would fundamentally change my life forever.

I'm not a 'God told me so' type person. I could count on my fingers the amount of times I have heard God speak in an almost audible way. But about 20 minutes from the little town of Cowra, I heard God speak in a simple, gentle way, and this is how it went. "Son", (Yes), "you know the love you felt for your daughter last night?" I knew that well. I would have given anything to stop her suffering. "Of course I do," I replied. Then His reply came as clear as crystal, in a phrase I will never forget. "I love you even more."

I cannot adequately tell you with words how that affected my life. God's words were so simple, yet so profound, that they rocked me and changed my perspective of God. Tears flooded from my eyes so much I literally couldn't drive. I pulled over and opened the door to let out the floodwater that was now pouring inside the car.

Before that day I had known God's love. You have read my story about how I met God and His love saved me and set me free. But that day I understood in a new depth God's love. Could it be that without my little girl's illness and the pain we all went through, that I may never have understood God's love in such a way? I don't know. What I saw as a thorn in the flesh of the whole family, God saw as a beautiful rose about to bloom.

That night, and many other nights, I would have done anything to stop my little girl's suffering. On the road to Cowra I realized the truth of God's love in the most tangible of ways. It's the reason for God's intervention into our world that first Christmas. He came because His message is that of a father who would do anything to stop His children's suffering. "I love you even more" He says to each of us today. I don't have the answer to all of human suffering, but I do know the answer while in human suffering.

Dr James Dobson, the Christian psychologist, observed that, "nothing is wasted in God's economy". That 'nothing' includes depression, anxiety and mental illness.

Mind over Mood, while not written from a Christian perspective, illustrates the possible benefits of depression thus:

"An oyster creates a pearl out of a grain of sand. The grain of sand is an irritant to the oyster. In response to the discomfort, the oyster creates a smooth, protective coating that encases the sand and provides relief. The result is a beautiful pearl. For an oyster, an irritant becomes the seed for something new."[6]

We have seen miracles in our daughter's life, and through her illness she has become an incredible carer of people with a soft heart toward the suffering of others.

---

6 D Greenberger & C Padesky, Mind over Mood, (New York: Guilford, 1995)

There is a guy in the Bible who suffered probably more than anyone else, and he makes a very interesting observation. His name is Job, and right at the end of the Book of Job in the Old Testament he makes a statement that is incredibly profound in its simplicity. In chapter after chapter we read of his suffering and heartache. Then after God has spoken, correcting him and his so-called friends that sat around him in his suffering, Job comes to a conclusion:

Job 42:5

My ears had heard of you, but now my eyes have seen you.

I can say with Job, that I have seen God. I have seen God in my little girls sickness; I have seen God in my personal battle with depression and mental illness. It is so much more than just hearing of Him, because when we see Him in and through our suffering, we are changed forever.

What is it that God would have you see Him more clearly through?

IN CHRIST

I have been where the Psalmist was:

Psalm 6:6

I am worn out from groaning; all night long I flood my bed with weeping and drench my couch with tears.

Try this today. Say with me, "I am valued by God". or, "My value is in God". or, "I am of great value just as I am to my God."

In the Bible we come across these two words together often—'*in Christ*'. God does not want us to live in a false understanding of our value to Him, nor in a state of always considering our lack of worth. Our value is not the sum of our achievements nor the sum of our failures. To understand our true value, the secret lies not in our efforts or in our mistakes. The secret lies '*in Christ*'. Let's look at some of the '*in Christ*' statements made in the scriptures:

Romans 8:1

Therefore, there is now no condemnation for those who are in Christ Jesus.

Romans 8:39

Neither height nor depth, nor anything else in all creation, will be able to separate us from the love of God that is in Christ Jesus our Lord.

1 Corinthians 15:22

So, in Christ, all will be made alive.

2 Corinthians 3:14

But their minds were made dull, for to this day the same veil remains when the old covenant is read. It has not been removed, because only in Christ is it taken away.

The verse directly above tells us that a veil remains upon people when the old ways of law are stated. But '*in Christ*' the veil is removed, causing us to go from not seeing clearly, to now, '*in Christ*', being able to see the wonders of God.

2 Corinthians 5:17

Therefore, if anyone is in Christ, he is a new creation; the old has gone, the new has come!

Galatians 3:26

Sons through faith 'in Christ'.

Paul understands where the value comes from:

Philippians 3:14

I press on toward the goal to win the prize for which

God has called me heavenward in Christ Jesus.

Philippians 4:19

And my God will meet all your needs according to his glorious riches in Christ Jesus.

Colossians 2:10

Given fullness 'in Christ'.

'*In Christ*', or out of Christ, we are still valued by Christ just as we are, created and loved by God. However, 'in Christ', we come under this divine protection of a loving heavenly father. Not just divine protection, but also divine provision.

GOD VALUES AND LOVES US

Let us get away from this whole idea of God being full of anger and wrath and realize the truth. God values and loves us, even in the state we are in, with an everlasting passion. Consider this for a moment. Even when Adam and Eve turned from God and were rebellious against Him, He still made them clothes, and cared for them as they left Eden.

YOUR NAME

The Bible says this:

Isaiah 49:1

Listen to me, you islands; hear this, you distant nations: Before I was born the LORD called me; from my birth he has made mention of my name.

Your name and my name were mentioned before our birth in eternity. It has been said that there may be accidental parents but there is no such thing as an accidental child.

Imagine this: a teenage girl and boy sleep together, she becomes pregnant and the young boy doesn't want this heavy responsibility, and leaves. The child is born to a single mother—and a very young one at that. This child can be seen as a mistake, and I see so many young people end up in very difficult circumstances because of poor decisions. Yet! This is where we need to stretch our minds; this child was still knitted together by God Himself, created in the miracle of birth and breathed into by God, so he or she could live. There is still a majestic plan in place for that child.

Isaiah 49:15-16 (MSG)

> *Can a mother forget the infant at her breast, walk away from the baby she bore? But even if mothers forget, I'd never forget you—never. Look, I've written your names on the backs of my hands. The walls you're rebuilding are never out of my sight.*

Knowing that from God's perspective, even if a mother can forget the child at her breast, God will never forget us, is fundamental to knowing our value.

What's God saying? He's saying, "Listen to me, I value you even higher than a mother values her new born child."

There is no doubt that, at its core, the Bible is truly the greatest love story ever told. There is separation, desperation and the love of God always seeking to find a way to reconcile people to Himself. Isn't this the gospel—God so loved each one of us, just as we are, that Jesus came into this world and went through so much pain and suffering to win us back?

This is the most amazing thing of all time, yet mankind seems to miss it. The thinking that God is all about wrath, lightning bolts, condemnation and anger is fundamentally wrong. Yes, he is a righteous and holy God, and wickedness will reap its own reward. This is why I believe if people realized how much God loves them, they would flock to Him. Not to religion, but to Jesus. It really is all about God's love and the value He places on each of us just because we are us!

Let's look at another passage in the Bible:

Luke 12:7 (MSG)

What's the price of two or three pet canaries? Some loose change, right? But God never overlooks a single one. And he pays even greater attention to you, down to the last detail—even numbering the hairs on your head! So don't be intimidated by all this bully talk. You're worth more than a million canaries.

JESUS' X-RAY VISION

Jesus had this ability to see through the outer layers and look at the value of every single individual as precious. This next passage is about a woman caught in the act of adultery, a crime punishable by death according to Jewish law.

John 8:2-11 (MSG)

Jesus went across to Mount Olives, but he was soon back in the Temple again. Swarms of people came to him. He sat down and taught them. The religion scholars and Pharisees led in a woman who had been caught in an act of adultery. They stood her in plain sight of everyone and said, "Teacher, this woman was caught red-handed in the act of adultery. Moses, in the Law, gives orders to stone such persons. What do you say?" They were trying to trap him into saying something incriminating so they could bring charges against him.

Jesus bent down and wrote with his finger in the dirt. They kept at him, badgering him. He straightened up and said, "The sinless one among you, go first: Throw the stone." Bending down again, he wrote some more in the dirt.

Hearing that, they walked away, one after another, beginning with the oldest. The woman was left alone.

Jesus stood up and spoke to her. "Woman, where are they? Does no one condemn you?"

"No one, Master."

"Neither do I," said Jesus. "Go on your way. From now on, don't sin."

Here we see an angry mob focused on a woman caught in sin. The full letter of the law would have had her stoned to death. She was guilty beyond doubt and had no way out. There are lots of lessons in this passage, but just look at the heart of Jesus here. Look at the posture of Jesus. He did not stand and in anger shout at this woman or tear shreds off her for her wrong doings. He bent down and started to write in the dirt. We don't know what He wrote, but we can see His heart for love over condemnation, as He places such a high value on this lady. He does not excuse her behavior but He looks beyond it to her value. This woman, caught in wickedness, was guilty and deserving death, yet Jesus saw her not as defined by her outward behavior but rather as a precious and valued person. We are all created special and valued in God's eyes.

Psalm 139:1-18

O LORD, you have searched me and you know me.

You know when I sit and when I rise; you perceive my thoughts from afar.

You discern my going out and my lying down; you are familiar with all my ways.

Before a word is on my tongue you know it completely, O LORD.

You hem me in—behind and before; you have laid your hand upon me.

Such knowledge is too wonderful for me, too lofty for me to attain.

Where can I go from your Spirit? Where can I flee from your presence?

If I go up to the heavens, you are there; if I make my bed in the depths, you are there.

If I rise on the wings of the dawn, if I settle on the far side of the sea,

even there your hand will guide me, your right hand will hold me fast.

If I say, "Surely the darkness will hide me and the light become night around me,"

even the darkness will not be dark to you; the night will shine like the day, for darkness is as light to you.

For you created my inmost being; you knit me together in my mother's womb.

I praise you because I am fearfully and wonderfully made; your works are wonderful, I know that full well.

My frame was not hidden from you when I was made in the secret place. When I was woven together in the depths of the earth,

your eyes saw my unformed body. All the days ordained for me were written in your book before one of them came to be.

How precious to me are your thoughts, O God! How vast is the sum of them!

Were I to count them, they would outnumber the grains of sand. When I awake, I am still with you.

This was one of the first passages I learnt as a new believer and, still to this day, it thrills my heart.

I wonder how many of us read this passage, yet don't really believe it? I don't think I really understood this until that day on the road to Cowra. I don't think we consciously say, "I don't believe that." However our thoughts and lives reflect that we don't.

I don't know about you, but my mirror would tell me that if I'm made in God's image, then God doesn't look too good. God created us, and then when we came to Him, He recreated us. The Bible tells us that He is in the process of changing us *'from glory to glory.'* **2 Corinthians 3:18 (KJV)** In this passage we see the hands of God forming our being and creating who we are; our DNA code, our personality traits, our gifts and abilities. Why would the God who cast the stars into the sky and who created a universe so great, that we humans with all our technologies cannot reach the end of it, choose to value us above all creation? I want you to try to fathom this one for a moment. The God who did all these things, creating billions of stars that are all under His control, would trade them *all* in for one of you! Just as you are! Medicated, messed-up, broken and emotionally bruised, just simply you!

As amazing as it is, given a choice of the entire universe with its wonders in one hand, or the person reading this book in the other, God will take you every time! That's the real value of you!

Romans 5:6-11 (MSG)

Christ arrives right on time to make this happen. He didn't, and doesn't, wait for us to get ready. He presented himself for this sacrificial death when we were far too weak and rebellious to do anything to get ourselves ready. And even if we hadn't been so weak, we wouldn't have known what to do anyway. We can understand someone dying for a person worth dying for, and we can understand how someone good and noble could inspire us to selfless sacrifice. But God put his love on the line for us by offering his Son in sacrificial death while we were of no use whatever to him.

Now that we are set right with God by means of this sacrificial death, the consummate blood sacrifice, there is no longer a question of being at odds with God in any way. If, when we were at our worst, we were put on friendly terms with God by the sacrificial death of his Son, now that we're at our best, just think of how our lives will expand and deepen by means of his resurrection life! Now that we have actually received this amazing friendship with God, we are no longer content to simply say it in plodding prose. We sing and shout our praises to God through Jesus, the Messiah!

We were a long way off! Our natural thinking would say that we were of not much value. Yet, and it's a huge Yet, Christ chose to sacrifice His greatness for our pathetic state, because He values us not for what we have accomplished, or our wealth and achievements. He values us because we are created by and loved by God. Whether we realize it or not, we are all children of God and valued this way.

SO WE'RE MESSED UP. WELCOME TO THE CLUB.

This passage in the Bible always makes me jump with happiness:

1 Corinthians 1:25-31

For the foolishness of God is wiser than man's wisdom and the weakness of God is stronger than man's strength.

Brothers, think of what you were when you were called. Not many of you were wise by human standards; not many were influential; not many were of noble birth. But God chose the foolish things of the world to shame the wise; God chose the weak things of the world to shame the strong. He chose the lowly things of this world and the despised things—and the things that are not—to nullify the things that are, so that no one may boast before him. It is because of him that you are in Christ Jesus, who has become for us wisdom from God—that is, our righteousness, holiness and redemption. Therefore, as it is written: 'Let him who boasts boast in the Lord.'

Why I love this passage so much is this; I qualify. So do you for that matter. It's not by natural selection, or by my wisdom and understanding. No, it's by God's grace and yes, I can boast. I can boast not in my self-sufficiency or abilities, although they are many, vast and extraordinary (just joking!), but in God's great love and grace He has placed on me.

THE VALUE OF YOU, AGAIN

1 Peter 1:18, 19 (NLT)

For you know that God paid a ransom to save you from the empty life you inherited from your ancestors. And the ransom he paid was not mere gold or silver. It was the precious blood of Christ, the sinless, spotless Lamb of God.

The value or price on us was huge. We cost a lot; we cost the sacrifice of God. Yet God was more than willing to pay the price for us.

The way we perceive our value affects our conduct. Can we do all things through Christ who gives us strength? Yes, I believe so. Can we reach a point where our lives are lived beyond depression and mental illness? Yes, I know so!

CHANGING THE DEFAULT SETTING

If we perceive our value as low, then everything we do in our lives comes from that low value setting. It's like a 'default setting' pre-programmed onto our hard drive which establishes our running systems responses.

For instance: A low self worth (an inner belief 'default setting'), will cause us to always be trying to prove our worth.

This was my 'default setting' for many years. Believing I was of little worth, I went about trying to prove to the world that I was of value. This was the deep motivation behind going into debt early in life to buy the status symbol car and the motivation behind the clothes I would wear. Everything was about somehow proving that what I deep down believed to be true was really not true. An even deeper setting is the one every human has on the planet—the setting that desires love. So powerful is this desire and God-given programming, that we will do anything to be loved or prove we are worthy of being loved and accepted.

When I realized that I was loved and accepted by God simply because of His greatness rather than my effort, it changed my life! That was a freedom day! That was when God changed the 'default setting'. I truly believe that just grabbing this fact will stop millions spiraling into depression. Recovery will become a reality rather than a pipe dream. Once the 'default setting' is reset to factor in our true value, everything changes. Oh, everything! The entire world changes color. Grays start to be overwhelmed by bright life-filled colors. Negativity starts to lose the battle as positive love comes into ascendancy. Striving and anxiety are conquered by peace. The fog lifts and the surrounding beauty is seen again. It's the place to live. You may have spent your entire life with the wrong 'default setting' controlling your actions and reactions. Choose today to see your true value, choose today to grasp this truth and hold it so tight that you will never let it go. If you find in life you are hanging by just one thing and it's this, then that is enough to hold you from falling!

The Ephesians didn't get it either. The Apostle Paul was trying to get his point across to the Ephesian believers. This group had so much of this world's natural possessions. They had lots of good things going for them, but were missing some vital understanding about who they actually were 'in Christ'.

Ephesians 1:16-23

For this reason, ever since I heard about your faith

in the Lord Jesus and your love for all the saints, I have not stopped giving thanks for you, remembering you in my prayers. I keep asking that the God of our Lord Jesus Christ, the glorious Father, may give you the Spirit of wisdom and revelation, so that you may know him better. I pray also that the eyes of your heart may be enlightened in order that you may know the hope to which he has called you, the riches of his glorious inheritance in the saints, and his incomparably great power for us who believe. That power is like the working of his mighty strength, which he exerted in Christ when he raised him from the dead and seated him at his right hand in the heavenly realms, far above all rule and authority, power and dominion, and every title that can be given, not only in the present age but also in the one to come. And God placed all things under his feet and appointed him to be head over everything for the church, which is his body, the fullness of him who fills everything in every way.

Ephesians 3:14-21

For this reason I kneel before the Father, from whom his whole family in heaven and on earth derives its name. I pray that out of his glorious riches he may strengthen you with power through his Spirit in your inner being, so that Christ may dwell in your hearts through faith. And I pray that you, being rooted and established in love, may have power, together with all the saints, to grasp how wide and long and high and deep is the love of Christ, and to know this love that surpasses knowledge—that you may be filled to the measure of all the fullness of God. Now to him who is able to do immeasurably more than all we ask or imagine, according to his power that is at work within us, to him be glory in the church and in Christ Jesus throughout all generations, forever and ever! Amen.

COMING HOME

In the third part of Luke 15, we see the story of the lost (prodigal) son.

Luke 15:11-24

Jesus continued: "There was a man who had two sons. The younger one said to his father, "Father, give me my share of the estate." So he divided his property between them.

Not long after that, the younger son got together all he had, set off for a distant country and there squandered his wealth in wild living. After he had spent everything, there was a severe famine in that whole country, and he began to be in need. So he went and hired himself out to a citizen of that country, who sent him to his fields to feed pigs, He longed to fill his stomach with the pods that the pigs were eating, but no one gave him anything.

When he came to his senses, he said, "How many of my father's hired men have food to spare, and here I am starving to death! I will set out and go back to my father and say to him: Father, I have sinned against heaven and against you. I am no longer worthy to be called your son; make me like one of your hired men." So he got up and went to his father. But while he was still a long way off, his father saw him and was filled with compassion for him; he ran to his son, threw his arms around him and kissed him.

The son said to him, "Father, I have sinned against heaven and against you. I am no longer worthy to be called your son." But the father said to his servants, "Quick! Bring the best robe and put it on him. Put a ring on his finger and sandals on his feet. Bring the fattened calf and kill it. Let's have a feast and celebrate. For this son of mine was dead and is alive again; he was lost and is found." So they began to celebrate.

Some thoughts on this passage:

How the son saw himself upon his return is interesting. He placed his value on the sum of his achievements, or in this case, his failure. In verse 19, when he said he was 'no longer worthy' he saw himself and his value or worth as lost due to his wasteful behavior. Where his behavior was wrong, and he wasted a huge amount living in a wrong way, his value was not in his failure or losses.

Too often we judge our worth by the circumstances of life. We look around us and assume our value is proportionate to life's status. This young man had failed. Remember, 'failure is an event, never a person'. He had found himself in a situation of starvation, and for a young Jewish man, the most desperate of positions as a pig-feeder. But this is a fact; he as a person was of the same value to God as he had ever been.

His father, who is parallel to our heavenly Father, saw the reality of the situation and the young man. Notice how the father never once said stuff like, "You look a mess, son," or, "You could have cleaned yourself up a bit." What about, "You wasted half my wealth, you idiot," or even, "I knew you'd mess it up; I told you so." In fact, we see nowhere that this young man's mistakes are even mentioned by the Father.

This young man was, and always will be a son of his father. We can take from this the fact that you and I, no matter our life's situations or faults and failings or our past, whether good or bad, are valued greatly by God simply because we are who we are.

The robe, the ring and the sandals in verse 22 are all symbols of the value the father placed on the son. These symbols show his value simply because of who he is, and not in anything he has done. I will use myself again as an example here because I can identify with this young man, and without going again into the before-knowing-Christ-Gary, I must admit that it took a long time for me to realize this fact. Quite often when we come to Christ, it is at a low point or a point of great challenge in life. This is common. As humans we tend to be self-sufficient and we only look to God when there is some form of crisis. After coming to Christ I still saw my value as the sum of who I had become. Realizing the truth of who we become in Christ is a vital part of the answer to this whole value question. I had tried and failed. Although I knew I was forgiven and that God loved me, and I was rejoicing in those facts, I still saw myself as pretty useless, and a failure. I was happy, loving God and filled with an amazing joy in my salvation. I was worshipping Him with my whole heart and mind, and loving my Savior with all I had. However, that deep belief of my own worth as simply me, was faulty. Now, if *I* spent years realizing this, I assume that others may struggle with it as well. I have watched many people (including myself) come to Christ and throw themselves into His service fully, yet never deal with that constant nagging and flawed belief system that cries out deep from within, "you're not worthy". This belief has a foundation of truth, yet can become a binding and limiting issue for so many if the realization of the fullness of Christ 'in' us is not grasped.

'IN CHRIST' IS THE ANSWER

When we realize that our value is great '*in Christ*', it changes everything. A Christ-follower, or not a Christ-follower, the fact that the creator of this universe knitted each of us together in our mother's womb and saw our unformed body shows us the value He places on each individual, simply because we are created by Him. Someone once said, "God don't make no junk", and that is so true.

I know I have repeated this many times in this chapter but I cannot understate its importance! Your value is in Christ's love for you. Your value is not in your accomplishments or wealth. It is in the fact that you are made and loved by God. Imagine how your world will change or how differently you will see this world if this understanding takes hold and your true value becomes your default setting for life. That's the foundation for the real life that God talks about in the Bible.

Look around you tonight. When the stars come out in the blackness of the sky, repeat those words God said to me that day on the lonely road, "I love you even more". He does!

WINNING BETWEEN THE EARS

STEP 4: CONTROLLING THE THOUGHT LIFE

The mind is an incredibly powerful thing. Our thoughts will affect every aspect of our lives.

It has been stated correctly: "We are either controlled by our thoughts, or we control our thoughts!"

I remember hearing a story of a pastor counseling a husband and wife who were about to be divorced. In a session where only the wife was present, she expressed that her husband was lazy, self-centered and inconsiderate. She wanted out, as he was not the man she thought she had married. The pastor advised her to spend the next month thinking of him and loving him as if he were the man she dreamed of being married to. Without her husband being aware of the advice, she started focusing on only his good points. Although it was a struggle at first, she proceeded for the next month to think and treat him that way. A month later the wife again sat in the pastor's office and he asked her, "So do you still want to get the divorce?" Her response was, "No, he's changed so much and I really love him." What brought about this change were the actions that flowed from a repatterning of the thought process.

In this chapter we are about to do some serious thinking about how we think.

Without doubt, this element of the process to achieve a life beyond depression and mental illness is the most exciting, challenging, and potentially life-changing thing than anything else in this book.

Understanding that we cannot separate thoughts from feelings, nor feelings from behaviors is vital in this process. They are interrelated, interdependent and intertwined because what we think affects how we feel, and what we think and feel affects our physical health. Our physical health can, and does, affect our thoughts and emotions. Our thoughts, feelings and physical health affect our actions and the subsequent results of these actions.

Within the holistic approach required for recovery from depression and mental illness is the vital element of how we treat and control our thought processes. We will be focusing our attention during this chapter on the area of our thought life. This will include the true and false thought patterning of our minds, how we think, and the patterning of our mind that dominates the way we think. Wrong or false thought patterning is the biggest contributor to depression. If we can learn to control and repattern our thought processes, it will be the greatest step we can take in our recovery.

When we are involved constantly in something that consumes us, whether it is good or bad, we can, in a sense, 'not see the forest for the trees'. For example, if I was to take on a work project that occupies large amounts of my time, and it seemed as though it was all I could think about—a bit like writing this book—being consumed with it means that other very important things could be missed. To have someone with an objective viewpoint come in and look at my situation can at times be very beneficial. Perhaps an observer or friend can come alongside me and say something to the effect of, "Hey Gary, you're really busy and you're doing a great job. Have you realized that your daughter seems to be trying to get your attention?" I may have missed the signs because of my preoccupation with the task at hand. This is so easy to do, especially if the task has a high mission attached to it. I become blind because of my consuming situation. This is why at times an independent observer, counselor, minister or friend can be a vital help in life's situations.

Being a male and loving sport, I can get very consumed by the TV coverage. Sometimes my children will say, "Dad, Dad," and have to say it many times before I even hear them. It's a bloke thing! Most of the times it's okay, unless it's, "Dad, I broke my leg," or something similar. But what if I'm so lost in my thoughts that I miss my 16 year-old desperately needing to talk to her father about what's happening in her life? I'm so consumed by the task at hand that I keep missing the signs, and eventually she shuts down—even when I ask what's wrong, all I get is the "nothing" response.

Probably the clearest example of this I have seen has been in the business community. Men and women who have worked long and hard to achieve success often become very financially successful, only to find their partner leaves them. "I just didn't see it coming", they may say, and they're 100 percent correct. They didn't see it, because their mind was consumed with other things.

As we move through this process of learning to control and repattern our thought processes, allow me to give you some observations that may hit home. As an independent observer, who has the benefit of having struggled with depression and mental illness for many years, hopefully I can point out some things within this chapter that will really help.

In his excellent paper entitled *Depression and the Christian*[7], Dr David P Murray makes this statement:

> "Perhaps the most obvious symptoms of depression are the unhelpful patterns of thinking, which tend to distort a depressed person's view of reality in a false and negative way, and so add to the depression or anxiety."

The Bible makes this statement:

Romans 12:2

Do not conform any longer to the pattern of this world, but be transformed by the renewing of your mind. Then you will be able to test and approve what God's will is—his good, pleasing and perfect will.

In Romans 12:2, it speaks of the 'pattern' of this world. Our thoughts and actions stem from the patterning of the mind.

YOUR PERSONAL SUPER COMPUTER

The mind is a patterning super computer. Look at driving, for example. After we have been driving for years, we don't even think about the processes. They are patterned into our minds and thoughts. We act and react from the patterning established when we learn to drive. One religious organization proudly makes a statement: "Give me a child until they are five, and we will have them always." Why do they say this? Because they have discovered, rightly or wrongly, that if they pattern the child's thought process repetitively for a number of years, that child will for the rest of their lives, unless it is consciously changed, act according to that patterning established within their mind. It is the same thing Hitler did in World War II with the patterning of the thought processes of the Hitler Youth program.

When it comes to our fight for a life beyond depression and mental illness, the re-patterning of our thought processes is

7 Dr. David P Murray. Depression and the Christian February 2008

essential.

For those suffering in any way from depression or mental illness, you will know the mind is extremely powerful and an uncontrolled mind is extremely devastating. Let me help you in the repatterning of how we think. Once our thoughts are re-patterned, it's like a fresh breeze that rushes in, pushing away and dispersing the fog.

WEAPONS, BATTLES AND WARFARE

The next passage literally saved my life over and over again. This passage talks of weapons, battles and a war. We can relate this directly to the fight we face in our minds every day.

Even if today you would regard yourself as not a Christ-follower, this advice will still work for you. Biblical wisdom is not limited to those who follow Christ. It certainly helps if you do trust God within this process and divine power enables quicker results.

2 Corinthians 10:3-5

> *For though we live in the world, we do not wage war as the world does. The weapons we fight with are not the weapons of the world. On the contrary, they have divine power to demolish strongholds. We demolish arguments and every pretension that sets itself up against the knowledge of God, and we take captive every thought to make it obedient to Christ.*

A FIGHT TO THE DEATH

Make no mistake; this is a fight, and it's a fight to the death. The Bible talks of waging war, and this is what we must do. The scriptures are not kidding around. It is hard to wage war, especially if the war for the mind seems to be lost or is heading that way. But just because there have been periods of defeat, it does not mean the war is lost.

This chapter is a war-winning strategy. It's not instant; it's not easy, but it is truth and the secret to victory.

Growing up, my mum and dad used all the 'older person' sayings. You know the ones. They are the things that you swear you would never say to your children and then do, like, "There's no such thing as a free lunch," and "Lose the attitude or you're not going anywhere." The list is endless. My dad's personal favorite: "Better out than in, I always say."

Moving right along.

What about this one: "Good things are worth fighting for." This victory over depression and mental illness is worth fighting for.

But who said that victory would be easy? However, victory is victory nonetheless, and we must fight for what is right. We must fight for our lives, our families and our relationships, and the fight is most fierce between our ears. We win this fight, and we win the war!

I'm a huge fan of the great orator, Winston Churchill. In Britain's darkest hours during World War II, he wrote speeches that inspired a nation that stood on the brink of destruction. I would like to take a few of his quotes regarding World War II and the fight for survival, and shine some light upon how we handle the war we fight within our minds. Churchill wrote regarding the air war over Britain:

'The flying peril is not a peril from which one can fly. We cannot possibly retreat. We cannot move London.'[8]

If we apply this principle to controlling our minds, we must realize that our thoughts are the flying peril that we cannot fly from, for we cannot move ourselves. So we must fight! Many people

---

8 House of Commons, 28th November 1934

do try to move themselves. We call it 'doing a geographical'. The thinking is that escape will provide the answer. I remember when I moved from Sydney back to Coffs Harbour, my mind came with me. Our minds go with us, so in reality we cannot run, we must fight!

VICTORY IN SPITE OF ALL TERROR

Another classic quote from the great man:

'Victory, victory at all costs, victory in spite of all terror, victory however long and hard the road might be; for without victory there is no survival.'

Understand this: there will be terror, and the road could be long and hard, but victory must be obtained because without victory, as Churchill puts it, 'There is no survival.'

My story is that victory is possible. Yes it took time, yes it was challenging, but is victory over depression, emotional and mental illness attainable? A resounding yes!

A MILITARY MINDSET

A military campaign requires strategy for success, so to be successful our campaign requires strategy towards our thoughts.

To surrender is not to survive, but rather to die within the concentration camps of our mind, slowly perishing from within our own thoughts.

Personally, I believe that one of the greatest tragedies of our time is that so many have given up. They believe the lie that things cannot change. They believe that they are somehow stuck in this place, due to a code implanted upon them that cannot change. Therefore, they exist in a semi-life, reinforcing their patterned thinking that life will not get better. Even if you have tried and fallen many times, stand again with me and I will, to the best of my ability, try to equip you, with God's help, to be able to stay standing.

We won't win every battle, but when we repattern our thinking, we will win the war.

WELCOME TO FIGHT CLUB

It is my desire throughout this chapter to speak into lives, and inspire the willingness to fight this good fight. To fight with all we have, then get up and fight again. In Ephesians chapter 6, Paul tells us that we are in this battle and to clothe ourselves with the armor of God. Read this passage with me as we launch into what I believe is the most liberating truth these pages hold.

Ephesians 6:10-17

Finally, be strong in the Lord and in his mighty power. Put on the full armor of God so that you can take your stand against the devil's schemes. For our struggle is not against flesh and blood, but against the rulers, against the authorities, against the powers of this dark world and against the spiritual forces of evil in the heavenly realms. Therefore put on the full armor of God, so that when the day of evil comes, you may be able to stand your ground, and after you have done everything, to stand. Stand firm then, with the belt of truth buckled around your waist, with the breastplate of righteousness in place, and with your feet fitted with the readiness that comes from the gospel of peace. In addition to all this, take up the shield of faith, with which you can extinguish all the flaming arrows of the evil one. Take the helmet of salvation and the sword of the Spirit, which is the word of God.

The first statement embodies how we can achieve victory within the lessons put forward in this chapter, 'and in *His* mighty power'. This is one of those verses that we should make into a fridge magnet so we can see it all the time and be reminded of 'His mighty power'. This statement may sound impossible to you, however it is not. Let us take steps to control our minds for the victory and betterment of ourselves and those around us.

'The battle for Europe has ended, and the battle for Britain has begun.'

Churchill made this observation after the fall of Europe. The world could see that Germany had taken the rest of Europe and that only Britain remained to stand against insurmountable odds. Let's remind ourselves of the outcome of World War II. Britain did not fall and the Allies won. They did not win every battle along the way, but they won the war! They won through determination and, I believe, some divine intervention as well. If you examine the supernatural weather conditions that helped save thousands during the Dunkirk evacuation and the channel crossings, it's clear prayers were being answered.

We will take the heavy bombardments and all that the enemy of our souls can throw at us. Expect it to happen and prepare for the onslaught. However, know this: victory will be attained! He who is for us is far greater than he who is against us!

Do we let the bombardment of our thoughts bring the destruction of our lives or do we choose today not to surrender, but fight with all that is within us by the 'power of His might' for this illusive, yet very real victory?

If you are a committed Christ-follower, you must realize that you are not alone in this fight. If we were alone we would not be able to stand. The enemy is too strong and the road too hard. Yet, in Christ's power we are able to stand and, after having done all, to still be standing. If at this stage you feel a long way from God or totally disillusioned by the whole church thing, I want to encourage you in something. Firstly, you are actually not far from Him at all, because He tells us in the Bible that He is 'closer than the breath we breathe.' Secondly, I want you to listen. Listen with your heart for Him to speak to you through these passages.

2 Corinthians 10:3-5 (MSG)

The world is unprincipled. It's dog-eat-dog out there! The world doesn't fight fair. But we don't live or fight our battles that way—never have and never will. The tools of our trade aren't for marketing or manipulation, but they are for demolishing that entire massively corrupt culture. We use our powerful God-tools for smashing warped philosophies, tearing down barriers erected against the truth of God, fitting every loose thought and emotion and impulse into the structure of life shaped by Christ. Our tools are ready at hand for clearing the ground of every obstruction and building lives of obedience into maturity.

WHAT IS A STRONGHOLD?

It is a fortified position that is not easy to overpower. When it comes to strongholds in our lives, let us adapt what we are talking about directly to these strongholds. I will use a few examples later. However, you know your strongholds better than I do, so apply these principles to your strongholds and remember that strongholds are not taken easily.

It's the divine power infusing the choices we make that will determine success in overcoming strongholds.

SOUND MIND OR SELF-DISCIPLINE?

2 Timothy 1:7 (KJV)

For God hath not given us the spirit of fear; but of power, and of love, and of a sound mind.

2 Timothy 1:7 (NLT)

For God has not given us a spirit of fear and timidity, but of power, love, and self-discipline.

This passage is actually more a call to live a certain way rather than some sort of heavenly zap from above to correct our minds. The passage puts forward that there is a life to be achieved that is calm and well-balanced through using self-control.

There are songs sung about this verse, and I have heard it thumped from the pulpit that God has given you a sound mind, so claim it in faith. There is an element of truth in this philosophy; however, it is not the whole truth. Let me explain. '*Love, power and a sound mind*' are the words used here. Remember that these words were not originally written in English. The word translated in the King James Bible as 'sound mind' is *sophronismos*, meaning a 'calling to soundness of mind through self-discipline and self-control'.

It is in the process of the self-discipline that the soundness of the mind is developed or recreated.

The balance needs to be restored and it is through the self-discipline and control of the mind's thoughts that this is achieved. This is why the theme of this chapter is 'Controlling the thought life'. It is one of the great secrets to a well-balanced and well mind.

A LINE IN THE SAND

To defeat our enemy we must know his movements. In the passage we just read about the armor of God we see that Paul instructs us to stand against the Devil's schemes. When it comes to knowing our enemy, let's face the facts; if the devil can have a person so caught in their mind that they live a defeated, hurt, and hurting-others existence, then he is happy. A believer caught in bitterness will stay on a self-destructive pattern and be totally ineffective. In fact, they will turn more people from God than to Him, and therefore the Devil rejoices in that, because he wins. Come on, let's not let him win. If he's been winning, it is time to draw a line in the sand and fight for the truth and victory.

In 2 Kings 6:8-17 we read a fascinating story in which we can see that, through God, we are able to recognize and know our enemies tactics.

2 Kings 6:8-17

Now the king of Aram was at war with Israel. After conferring with his officers, he said, 'I will set up my camp in such and such a place.'

The man of God sent word to the king of Israel: 'Beware of passing that place, because the Arameans are going down there.' So the king of Israel checked on the place indicated by the man of God. Time and again Elisha warned the king, so that he was on his guard in such places.

This enraged the king of Aram. He summoned his officers and demanded of them, 'Will you not tell me which of us is on the side of the king of Israel?'

'None of us, my lord the king', said one of his officers, 'but Elisha, the prophet who is in Israel, tells the king of Israel the very words you speak in your bedroom.'

'Go, find out where he is', the king ordered, 'so I can send men and capture him.' The report came back: 'He is in Dothan.' Then he sent horses and chariots and a strong force there. They went by night and surrounded the city.

When the servant of the man of God got up and went out early the next morning, an army with horses and chariots had surrounded the city. 'Oh, my lord, what shall we do?' the servant asked.

'Don't be afraid', the prophet answered. 'Those who are with us are more than those who are with them.'

And Elisha prayed, 'O LORD, open his eyes so he may see.' Then the LORD opened the servant's eyes, and he looked and saw the hills full of horses and chariots of fire all around Elisha.

We see that the man of God was able to know the movements of the enemy. In my early years of battling with this, I had to learn a few things, and the learning only came through the power of God to help me. What was the one thing that the enemy wanted to happen to me? If you've read my story, it was obviously to take me back into a state of a wild uncontrolled mind. For me, it was to fall back into the old patterning of my thoughts and be lost in them, thus making me consider that Christ did not have the power to overcome the darkness of my mind. This would have resulted in a powerless and ineffective half-walk of stumbling with God and perhaps limping into heaven after years of mental anguish. Paul's prayer to the Ephesians church was '*that the eyes of your hearts may be opened.*' **Ephesians 1:18** Open to what? His desire was that their hearts may be open to the incredible wonders of God and who they had become.

Our hearts need to be open to the reality of this battle for our mind. Thankfully there is another wonderful thing in that passage that is worthy of noting. The servant of Elisha the prophet came out and, with his natural eyes, saw this huge army surrounding him and was fearful. But see this: the answer is not found in our natural eyes, but rather our spiritual understanding. Elisha prayed that the eyes of the fearful one would be opened, and he saw, for the first time, the heavenly army surrounding and protecting them. Oh, that's my prayer today—for your eyes to be opened to see. The forces may amass around us, and the enemy may try every dirty scheme to fill us full of fear, but know this: *'Greater is he who is within us, than he who is in the world.'* **1 John 4:4**

God is bigger and stronger than the darkest of darkness. There is enough light in God's little finger to brighten our darkest places.

THE WEIRDNESS OF 'THOUGHT PLAY'

This fight can be an everyday fight. Everybody has crazy thoughts. However, one of the dangers of people who tend to live in their minds is that they play with thoughts that are unhealthy. The weird thing is the sense of pleasure that at times this produces. Some thoughts give a false sense of pleasure, like a bitter person planning revenge gets a sense of fulfillment in the plotting. It's sort of sick I know, but in reality, being depressed or mentally ill is being sick. That is before guilt, bitterness, unforgiveness, and a myriad of other things happen as these thoughts become destructive.

THINKING ON THINKING

Let us take a look at thinking. I am sure most people go through life not considering the fact that we actually can gain control of our thought life.

In this world there are three main types of thinking:

1. Carnal thinking, which is anti-God thinking

2. Natural thinking

3. Spiritual thinking

Some may say I've forgotten a category; the people that simply don't think! I have known quite a few of them, and have been one myself many times. They are a category of their own, but seeing how they don't think and we are talking about thinking, we will simply leave them out and they won't be any the wiser! Certainly no one reading this book would fit into that category anyway.

My assumption is that if you have come this far on our journey together, then we will not have to deal with the 'carnal or anti-God' thinking. So I would like to spend a little time on the difference between 'natural' thinking and 'spiritual' thinking.

Natural thinking is what we do naturally and places our wisdom as the supreme guiding light. Spiritual thinking, on the other hand, is drawn from placing God's Word and God's wisdom as the highest source of guidance for our lives. I am not talking about sinful thinking. I genuinely believe that if you are reading this book, then your desire is for the things of God in your life. When I talk about spiritual thinking, I'm not talking about those people who are what I call 'weird Christians'—the ones who think that carpet can be demon-possessed, and if their washing machine breaks down they're under attack from the devil. You know them... so heavenly minded, that they are of no earthly use.

If you're still with me, let's keep going.

The Bible says this: '*When things are tough, consider, or think about things*'. **Ecclesiastes 7:14** This literally means that when times are tough, things are not going well and life is difficult, step back and consider. Consider things with a thought process that allows God into the picture.

IMAGINATION AND CONTROLLING THE THOUGHT LIFE

Even prophets of God have been known to mess this one up.

Ezekiel 13:2

> *Son of man, prophesy against the prophets of Israel who are now prophesying. Say to those who prophesy out of their own imagination: 'Hear the word of the LORD!'*

It's the divine power to control our thoughts that is required for the destroying of these strongholds within our minds. Remember the truth in this that a stronghold is by definition not something easy to prevail against. We may have had uncontrolled thought processes for years, and these thought processes, or the patterning of the mind, will not be changed overnight. These patterns will also seek to dominate and defend their stronghold. This is where we need the hand of God through His divine power to overcome.

The Bible says, '*Hear the Word of the Lord*' **Isaiah 66:5**. The answer to the imaginations and false thought patterning or processes is to come and 'hear the Word of the Lord'. It is not an instant quick fix, nor some new age, self-help philosophy, but rather a divine help reality. The Bible describes God as '*our help in time of need*'. Hebrews 4:16

I went for a walk down the beach this morning. Robyn and I strolled along and, at times, held hands. We looked into each other's eyes. The sea was flat and dolphins played in the crystal waters just off shore. It was beautiful. This type of scene could have been described as a 'perfect day.' But the discipline of controlling our mind does not start within the ease of nice feelings and pleasant breezes blowing across the green, rolling hills of our life. It doesn't begin with the warm, winter sun as we stroll down the beach, arm in arm, whispering sweet nothings in each other's ears. It is more like a howling gale through a narrow, shadowed canyon with sheer, unclimbable cliffs towering above on each side, where we begin to learn the discipline of controlling our mind. If you like the water analogy, it's not dolphins frolicking but rather sharks circling. Forget the sharks for a while and let's use the valley idea, because that fits the next scripture verse I want to use.

VALLEYS OF VICTORY

Note this as we go through: it is in the valley of the shadow of death that the strength of God is made evident.

Psalm 23:4

'Even though I walk through the valley of the shadow of death, I will fear not evil, for you are with me.'

It was not until King David walked within the dark valley that he could cry out like this to his God. In this valley, these ten simple words could be sung to God. Contained in these words is a lesson learned in the depth of a dark valley: 'I will fear no evil, for you are with me.' Notice how in the valley David did not confess God's presence to us with words like, 'for God is with me.' No, he spoke not about God but *to God*. 'For You are with me.' Dark valleys can be very cold and scary; nevertheless, these are the places of miracles.

There are a few things to note in this passage: There are 'valleys of the shadow of death', and we all, at times, will walk through them.

David shifted his focus from the valley, to the God who is bigger than any valley. This is, in effect, the controlling of a thought process.

He states that he is walking through the valley, not sitting or staying in it. He is not denying the valley or even trying to prove that, doctrinally, valleys don't exist for him. He owns where he is, who he is, and also who is there with him in the valley.

If it's depression, bi-polar disorder, anxiety attacks or any other mental illness, let's own the fact that it is a valley and it's dark. Don't deny it. It's like a leprous person saying, "I don't have leprosy"; that's just lying to ourselves. Also, own the fact that although this valley floor may be damp, dark, and cold, there is a way through the valley. It is not a dead end, so the valley is a temporary location, not a permanent residence. Don't confuse the temporary with the permanent.

In the power of the thought life is the power for change. In fact, I'm convinced that all positive change begins within the thought life. The thoughts of the valley and the pain in the valley can consume and draw a person into depths of despair. However, controlling your thinking within the valley is where the victory will begin to be won.

CHOOSING THE FOCUS

Consciously changing the focus of our thought is the key to unlocking this. This is not an automatic function of the mind as the mind will automatically run to its existing patterned responses. It will take conscious determination of thought. The mind will run to a patterned response, to a set of stimuli. Now, if our patterned response to difficulties in life is to let our mind control our emotions and thought processes in a negative, downward spiral, then unless conscious thought is introduced to the equation, the result will always be a patterned response leading to a destructive thought process.

Like a river, it will always flow the course of less resistance; that's what water does and that's what our minds do also. The prepatterned responses are the natural course or the least resistant. If we want to change the course of a river, we must resist the flow of its normal direction at the same time as creating a new pathway for it to flow through. In other words, we need to, in our mind, resist the prepatterned responses and create a new pathway for our thought processes to take.

There is a saying that goes like this:

"If we always do what we have always done, we will always get what we've always got."

In fact, a definition of insanity is:

"To continue doing the same thing, and expecting a different result."

The river will always flow the way of least resistance.

I remember for a long time as a believer, and a committed one at that, feeling so guilty because I would get these crazy thoughts even in the middle of great worship services. I'd have to cry out, begging God for forgiveness for my thoughts. It took me a while to figure out that God already knows my thoughts anyway. They don't surprise Him at all. In fact, maybe He has even had the same thoughts–as He is touched with the feelings of our weaknesses the Bible tells us.

You mean to say Jesus had thoughts that troubled Him? Yes, I think so. We know He was 'sorrowful unto death', that He got angry with people in the temple and knocked their tables over. He constantly tore shreds off the religious leaders for their hard-heartedness.

A REALITY ZAP

Many may cry, "I wish God would just zap my mind and fix it all." Sorry to disappoint on this one, but it doesn't work that way.

But God's way is better, we will see!

RE-PATTERNING

It is the repatterning of our thought processes that will bring about freedom. Rather than think of the valley, turn your thoughts consciously toward the One who is guiding you through the valley, to a place beyond the darkness of these places. This will be hard at first. Actually, this will probably be one of the most difficult things you will ever do. However, it will be one of the most rewarding. Our prepatterned responses will automatically kick in unless we consciously intervene. This is where a pre-emptive strike is truly worthwhile.

David said, "though I walk *through,*" not, "as I stay in."

He pre-emptively decided that this valley would be walked through, not lived in. Although life was lived within the valley for a time, it became part of the journey rather than the end destination. One of the great strengths of David's life, and we can read it in the Psalms, is his willingness while in the dark places of life, to turn his thoughts towards God who he knew loved and cared for him.

Here lies the difference between 'natural' and 'spiritual' thinking. If we look at natural thinking, it is precisely that—natural. It takes no effort! It sees with the natural eyes and will always focus on the darkness of the valley.

On the other hand, spiritual thinking takes effort. This is why many don't bother with it, and they exist in a semi-fulfilled state of frustrated Christianity. They know enough of the truth to be convicted, yet fall short of the liberty of being set free by it.

When the Bible tells us to renew our minds, it literally means to change our thinking and to repattern the prepatterned thought processes. It is the repatterning of our thought processes that will bring about the resulting freedom.

This statement is so true: "Change the way you think, you change your life." Or, "*as a man thinks, so is he.*"

Approaching our thoughts in a pre-emptive, proactive way rather than a purely reactive way means we become intentional on how we choose to think.

Our thinking will either:

Hinder us or help us

Lynch us or launch us

Cause us to stumble, or strengthen us to stand

Bind us or build us.

1 Corinthians 2:14 (NLT)

But people who aren't spiritual can't receive these truths from God's Spirit. It all sounds foolish to them and they can't understand it, for only those who are spiritual can understand what the Spirit means.

1 Corinthians 2:14

The man without the Spirit does not accept the things that come from the Spirit of God, for they are foolishness to him, and he cannot understand them, because they are spiritually discerned.

God has not called us to be ordinary natural thinkers, but rather extraordinary spiritual thinkers.

A very dear friend of mine—we walked the walk together for many years—is a notorious natural thinker. To give an example, he decided that his children needed part-time work in their later years of school. This is a great idea as it teaches them about money and work ethic and so on. Natural thinking says, "Well, they need work, so whatever the hours the employer gives them, they must do." The end result was that these amazing children, after being encouraged through natural thinking, ended up working when they needed to be in fellowship with other young people around church and in youth activities. The end result was they made money, yet died spiritually to the point of walking away from God and progressively destroying their lives. Spiritual thinking still would have pursued work, but given the spiritual development of these children the higher priority. It was not purposefully evil or anti-God thinking, just natural, unspiritual thinking. This friend of mine loved God and still does, yet still thinks in very natural, non-spiritual ways regarding the things of God. It is a very high price for incorrect thinking.

STINKIN' THINKIN'

Ephesians 4:17

So I tell you this, and insist on it in the Lord, that you must no longer live as the Gentiles do, in the futility of their thinking.

One of the greatest stories in the Bible regarding natural thinking is told in the gospel of Luke.

Luke 12:16-21 (NASB)

And He told them a parable, saying, 'The land of a rich man was very productive.' And he began reasoning to himself, saying, 'What shall I do, since I have no place to store my crops?' 'Then he said, 'this is what I will do: I will tear down my barns and build larger ones, and there I will store all my grain and my goods.' And I will say to my soul, 'Soul, you have many goods laid up for many years to come; take your ease, eat, drink and be merry.'

But God said to him, 'You fool! This very night your soul is required of you; and now who will own what you have prepared?'

So is the man who stores up treasure for himself, and is not rich toward God.

Having been involved in business and the sales and success industry for a large amount of my life, I find this a fascinating passage. What this man did made perfect sense to the natural mind. We would refer to him as a successful and wise business man, and he would be looked up to by many seeking natural wealth. We would have had him giving seminars and training programs. In reality his wealth was not the problem. His natural thinking was the problem. We could argue that the only reason he received such a great crop was 'the blessing of the Lord' in the first place, after all, the Bible tells us, *'the blessing of the Lord makes rich.'* **Proverbs 10:22**

The problem was never the riches, the problem was his poor state spiritually before God. His thoughts never turned to how this great blessing could benefit others. It was all about him. One sure way to tell if you're a natural thinker is to look at who you think about most of the time.

If it's you, then chances are very good that you're a natural thinker.

Another example was a person I knew many years ago. Before I met him, others had told me what a godly man he was. I became a believer through a Pentecostal church so people 'functioning in the spirit' would bring messages from the Lord and prophecies. About this man, people said things like; "When he brings a prophecy, it's like God is there, he speaks with such anointing." Now this is one of the saddest cases I have seen, as this man was a lovely man who loved God and without doubt meant well in all he did.

What had happened is he had gone into business; in fact, several businesses and God had blessed him. I've been in business and have seen the 'blessing of the Lord', and it is a good thing. However, there is a line that is crossed and although I cannot say where exactly this happens , it occurs when the thing that was meant for our good and the good of others becomes something that causes the opposite effect in our lives. I have seen this happen a few times when the so called 'blessing' is the very thing that draws a person from God and kills them spiritually. I think it is when the 'natural mind' takes over and things are not spiritually discerned. This man was so 'blessed' that his work would take him away from fellowship. That is always a sign that the 'blessing' has gone beyond where God intended because it becomes contrary to scripture. The work came in and it needed to be done on Sunday. Sundays became another work day and gathering together with God's people became secondary. Gradually, ever so gradually, this godly man died spiritually, drowning in what his natural mind perceived as 'blessing'.

In the positive, I've seen people like my brother-in-law Michael and his family throw in great paying positions to move to a third world country. Natural thinking... crazy! Yet they returned home after an extended trip, wealthier in a spiritual realm than they ever were naturally.

HOW I SEE ME, NATURALLY

Spiritually discerned thinking is a great key to obtaining a life beyond depression, emotional instability and mental illness. What do I mean?

Let us just consider how we actually see ourselves, and some decisions we can make that result from a natural method of thinking. This affects every aspect of our lives from finances to relationships to decision making. Let's just look at a few examples briefly.

'I'm really down today.'

Natural thinking says: I'll stay at home and not attend the church, life group or the family BBQ.

Result: This will lead to self dislike and even self loathing, through guilt and shame and looking at ourselves through the 'I'm not good enough' glasses. Remember; this will become a patterned response, thus producing a repeated action.

Spiritual thinking says: I know I don't feel like facing people, but I know it is probably the best thing for me to be around other believers and be in a positive environment, so I will go. So many know this, and at the point of going, they get the whole 'feeling unworthy' thing happening and stop. Yet if they go;

Result: The result could be an amazing breakthrough. I've had people say things like, "I was not going to come today, but I did, and God really touched me."

I love this because that person has shown that they are living with at least some spiritual discernment. It's the meeting that you don't want to be at that is more than likely the one you need to be at.

Giving to the local church

Natural thinking says: It's my money. I don't think I should give; churches are only after your money. Anyway, I need it, I worked hard for that.

Result: The frustration, the miserable feeling whenever the offerings are received in a service. Bitterness, greed and the scrooge mentality that is very destructive.

After all God says:

Proverbs 11:24 (NASB)

There is one who scatters, and yet increases all the more, and there is one who withholds what is justly due, and yet it results only in want.

Spiritual thinking says: Generosity is a mark of a believer in Christ and I choose from my conscious mind to give. Spiritual thinking sees the God element in the equation.

Result: Positive faith and an abundant life built upon a kingdom mindset.

It will be our mindset towards what we go through that will make the difference, rather than what we actually go through.

Isaiah 55:8-9

"For my thoughts are not your thoughts, neither are your ways my ways," declares the LORD.

As the heavens are higher than the earth, so are my ways higher than your ways and my thoughts than your thoughts.

If this is true (and seeing how God said it, we can assume it is) why then do we at times think that our natural way of thinking is wiser than His?

Let's face the facts here. If we determine to go on living with natural thinking as our guide, we can never fully reach beyond depression or mental illness, remembering that to go on thinking naturally will come naturally. If I am going to choose my wisdom over God's Word, then I should just as well shut the book now because it will not work. Besides, if our own thinking resulted in the mess we are in, then how stupid is it to think that our own natural thinking will get us out?

PATTERNING OUR MINDS

Bearing in mind that repetition is regarded as the way to master learning, let us continue. Our minds will form patterned reactions and responses to differing situations. These patterned responses usually come from a set of core beliefs about ourselves.

In a sense we are all self-fulfilling prophesies. It's our patterned mindsets that filter our thoughts, followed by our actions that lead directly to the results we obtain in life. This results in our thinking being reinforced, and the process continuing to determine the results of our lives. This is one of the reasons I detest hearing a parent or teacher say to a child that they are hopeless. For a start, it's a lie, and what it does to the psyche of that young person, is to begin or to reinforce a pattern of belief. A child that is told this often enough will adopt his hopelessness as a truth, and this mindset (or patterned thinking) will cause everything they touch to be tainted or filtered by that false belief until they genuinely believe that they are not good enough. The results will just reinforce this thought and consequently influence further behavior on a continual spiral downward. But it can change! It will take time, and depending upon the length of time, and the depth of the destructive patterning, these factors will influence the repatterning process. This is literally renewing the mind.

This, however, does work in a positive way as well. It just takes more effort. Some call this the 'Pygmalion effect', others the 'self-fulfilling prophecy effect'. The 'Pygmalion effect' comes from the ancient story of a sculptor named Pygmalion who set himself to create a statue of the ideal woman. He created this perfect woman and named her Galatea. She was so beautiful that he fell in love with his work of art. Such was his belief in his sculpture that he begged the goddess Aphrodite to breathe life into her. This the goddess did, and they all lived happily ever after, as any good fairy tale should end.

His belief brought about a reality. His belief influenced his actions to produce the resulting reality. You may know the Pygmalion story better through the movie *My Fair Lady.* In this movie Professor Higgins claims he can take a cockney flower girl and turn her into a duchess. In the end, they came to the realization that it was not the things that young Eliza Doolittle learnt that made the difference, but rather the way she was treated. It's interesting to note that the way she was treated established a set of patterns which her mind turned into beliefs, and thus changed and repatterned her thinking and her behavior, and the result followed. Again, we see that the results we desire follow directly from our thinking and perceptions. Most people who suffer from depression and mental illness genuinely desire freedom from their illness. I know I did, and I know that it was vital that the repatterning took place for my freedom.

In the sales industry I have been involved in the training of many successful sales people, as well as many that, sadly, have not made it. It is so interesting to note that it is not skill that will determine their success. I have watched incredibly gifted men and women come through the sales training. They have been given great tools to succeed yet these people still fall far short of what their gifting or ability would suggest is possible. Even if they do succeed moderately, there is something in them that seems to sabotage their success.

On the other hand, I have seen many who have come with very little in the way of skill and many who could not even speak English and these people have gone on to be great success stories.

This puzzled me, and if I'm honest, frustrated me no end, until one thing about these both sets of individuals stood out. It was this; the ones who became successful, for some reason had within them an inner belief that they could achieve success. It was not self-motivation hype. It was a core patterned sense of belief that governed their actions. On the other hand, I observed that many of these great and gifted people who were unsuccessful, or only achieved moderately, had somewhere within them a patterned belief that they couldn't reach beyond. I got to the point of looking for what I would call the 'underlying negative'.

One such person, who I once described as one of my closest friends, fitted this pattern. He had, and still does, have more talent in his little finger than I have in total. He was gifted in communication, and one of the most 'naturally gifted' sales people I have ever met. Yet in him was a patterned belief system that he couldn't rise above. He would do so much so well, yet his thoughts would trip him up all the time. The result is a man who, probably all his life, will be an incredibly gifted underachiever.

The patterning is faulty and why, we may not know. It could have been his childhood, his marriage, the environment he lived in or even a natural tendency. Whatever caused the patterning doesn't matter. It's the changing or repatterning that counts.

I personally battled with this for many years. You read the first few chapters of this book. My mind had been patterned with a false belief that I was hopeless and doomed to failure, through no one's fault, just circumstances. My constant sickness and dyslexia would have influenced these beliefs.

Now here is a secret. The battle for my life, my mind, my sanity, strength, hope, future, family, wife, children, friends and ministry—all of this was rescued by the repatterning of my thought processes into line with God's word.

CHOOSING TO REPATTERN

There is a choice in this. The choice is to repattern or not. It was no one else's choice but mine, as it is yours.

I'm a huge distance from being perfect, but I do live a life beyond depression and mental illness today because of this repatterning process.

Henry Ford once said:

"If you think you can, or if you think you cannot, you're right."

Proverbs 23:7 (NASB)

For as he thinks within himself, so he is.

This is why we must bring our thinking in line with God's Word. God's Word is *His* printed way of thought.

So how do we repattern our thinking? I'm glad you asked!

2 Corinthians 10:3-5

For though we live in the world, we do not wage war as the world does. The weapons we fight with are not the weapons of the world. On the contrary, they have divine power to demolish strongholds. We demolish arguments and every pretension that sets itself up against the knowledge of God and we take captive every thought to make it obedient to Christ.

The process of taking every thought captive can be challenging, but it is vital for recovery.

This is the first step in repatterning our thought processes. When someone is arrested and taken captive, the process is to hold them in custody until their guilt or innocence is proven against a set of charges and certain evidence. If the person is proven innocent, then they are freed, however, if the evidence proves them guilty, they are dealt with accordingly. Now don't get me wrong here. I am not advocating capital punishment for criminals. However I am advocating capital punishment for destructive thought patterns that cause endless suffering within lives.

For example; a thought comes into my mind. Now understand this: we will always get random thoughts. Let us use a thought regarding a past mistake. This is a good example because we all qualify for having made mistakes. If you're reading this book and you don't think you have ever made a mistake, I'm sorry but I cannot help you. We have all made mistakes. The thought may be regarding financial issues that caused hurt to people, or relational mistakes that cause a divided family, or a sin we once committed that even the thought of it sickens our stomachs. The list would be endless. So, the thought arrives, and 'bang' it's there. All of a sudden a wild thought in the middle of a beautiful worship service. What do we do now? I've had these thoughts and battled with them for years. I had 'you're worthless' thoughts whenever I was on a high place. Some of the downright wicked thoughts were so left field they would shock me.

What do we do? First; take it captive. Don't deny it or avoid it. Just grab it, and metaphorically place it in a holding cell. Don't play with it, just throw it in and lock it up. Then weigh the evidence. Let us just say I lied about something and that lie caused offence, as someone else took the punishment for something I did. Yet, this happened years ago, I have apologized to God, to the people involved, and tried to make amends for my lie.

So, this thought with the associated guilt arrives in my mind and I take it captive. Now, the Bible says to '*take captive every thought to make it obedient to Christ.*' **2 Corinthians 10:5** Being 'obedient to Christ' means to bring that thought into judgment in relation to what God's Word says. The Bible tells us that if we repent and turn from our sins, He is faithful and just to forgive all our mistakes and to cleanse us completely. So if I have repented, and thus turned from my lying ways and have been forgiven, then that thought is judged and condemned to the firing squad as irrelevant and false. For in Christ, '*though my sins were like scarlet, they are now whiter than snow*', **Isaiah 1:18** the Bible tells me. It is then time to shoot that thought for the fraud it is. Now, that thought may pester me for awhile, but continually shooting it down with what Christ says will eventually destroy its power over me.

SOUNDS HARD? OH YEAH!

If that sounds like hard work, well, yes it can be, but as we repattern our thinking to handle our thoughts like this, it will become easier and we will find ourselves living free from these old hindrances of the mind.

What about this example? Someone has done something that has caused me offence. It hurt me, and I'm still angry with them for what they have done. The thoughts regarding the offence come flooding in and carry with them all the hurts, bitterness and anger. So what do I do with that? My natural mind may say, 'I cannot forgive them for what they did, I will not forgive them, and I refuse' bearing in mind I cannot change what has happened.

This brings about a dilemma, as it has been proven that unresolved hurt, and living in a state of bitterness and unforgiveness, will generally lead to mental instability, anxiety and sickness. What do we do? Now this is huge for so many, and I will cover forgiveness a little later, but let us consider briefly these thoughts right now. Using the scripture we used in the first example, I must bring these thoughts into captivity, putting them in the 'lock up' or 'holding cell' and placing them on trial. Then, bringing these thoughts under the obedience of Christ, ask the question; is it right to keep this thought, or to shoot it for the lie it is?

LOOKING THE RIGHT DIRECTION

So many times, especially in the early years, the only thing that saved me was the choice not to live in my hurts, but rather, to fix my eyes on the goodness of God.

This is not something that can be achieved through our natural minds and thought processes. This is spiritually discerned, a repatterning that can only be achieved through the power of Christ in us.

The fixing of our eyes on the right thing during this process is again a vital step.

The Bible tells us:

Philippians 4:8 (NLT)

And now, dear brothers and sisters, one final thing. Fix your thoughts on what is true, and honorable, and right, and pure, and lovely, and admirable. Think about things that are excellent and worthy of praise.

One thing I have learned: when there is nothing in life worthy of praise except God—that's enough!

Philippians 4:8 (MSG)

Summing it all up, friends, I'd say you'll do best by filling your minds and meditating on things true, noble, reputable, authentic, compelling, gracious—the best, not the worst; the beautiful, not the ugly; things to praise, not things to curse. Put into practice what you learned from me, what you heard and saw and realized. Do that, and God, who makes everything work together, will work you into his most excellent harmonies.

A FINAL THOUGHT ON THINKING

In John 9:1-3, the Bible tells this amazing account of the healing of a man born blind.

John 9:1-3 (NASB)

As He passed by, He saw a man blind from birth. And His disciples asked Him, 'Rabbi, who sinned, this man or his parents that he would be born blind?'

Jesus answered, "It was neither that this man sinned, nor his parents; but it was so that the works of God might be displayed in him."

Could it be that your illness, my illness, and the depression, anxiety or mental illness of anyone who suffers this way could be there so that the work of God might be displayed in them?

I'm not saying that God caused it, but let us consider that God can use it.

Maybe not right now, but in the process, even the mentally ill can be beautiful in their time. I wonder about this passage because this man had been blind for a long time. For more than 40 years he had suffered from blindness, at a time when his blindness destined him to live a life of begging and mistreatment. The disciples wanted to attribute blame, as we tend to do being human. But Jesus said that no matter what caused his blindness, God would use it to bring about the display of God's greatness.

I can see now that all through my depression, anxiety, mental illness and the subsequent recovery process, God has been turning it all into a life that shows His great might.

Matthew 22:37

Jesus replied: "Love the Lord your God, with all your heart, and with all your soul, and with all your mind".

The Collins dictionary refers to the mind as 'the entity responsible for individual thought pattern'. So we can see that loving the Lord God with 'our entire mind' is to set the patterning of our minds around God.

Continually consciously placing our mind on God rather than the given situation of the life we are in, will begin the repatterning process. Eventually, the patterned responses will become constructive, based 'in Christ', rather than destructive, based on our own thoughts.

The Apostle Paul to the Philippians church makes an interesting statement:

Philippians 3:19-20

Their destiny is destruction, their god is their stomach, and their glory is in their shame. Their mind is on earthly things. But our citizenship is in heaven. And we eagerly await a Savior from there, the Lord Jesus Christ.

Those destined for destruction have their minds fixed on earthly things. Believers who have come to Christ, and been forgiven, know, or should know, that they are set for eternity. However, so many walk unknowingly into the destruction of their lives, their families and relationships because their minds are on earthly things. Refusing to see God and His mighty love working within our lives is to have our minds set on earthly things, and thus, to bring about the destruction of ourselves emotionally and mentally. Transformation only comes through the power of God.

Ephesians 1:17-19

I keep asking that the God of our Lord Jesus Christ, the glorious Father, may give you the Spirit of wisdom and revelation, so that you may know him better. I pray also

> *that the eyes of your heart may be enlightened in order that you may know the hope to which he has called you, the riches of his glorious inheritance in the saints, and his incomparably great power for us who believe. That power is like the working of his mighty strength,*

May our hearts be open to the truth of this knowledge. Let the God of all creation enlighten our hearts. As our hearts are enlightened, so our lives shall be lightened as well.

There is no sugar-coated way of saying this differently. It will take a determination, even a pig-headed determination to overcome these mental and emotional issues. It's a fight and a battle that needs to be won.

Choosing 'spiritual thinking' rather than 'natural thinking' begins the repatterning of our thoughts, taking every thought into captivity, and bringing it into obedience with the word of God. Doing this constantly until the mind is repatterned and our thoughts grow out of constructive patterning rather than destructive.

In this, the miraculous is accomplished.

LET'S GET PHYSICAL, PHYSICAL

STEP 5: WORKING OUT A WAY FORWARD

If you read this chapter title and are suddenly transported to seeing Olivia Newton John complete in workout gear, purple tights, sweat bands and leg warmers, then I'm with you. If not, YouTube 'Let's get physical Olivia Newton John' and you will soon learn.

We are going to look at the effects of physical activity in the recovery from depression and mental illness. If you're reading this book then chances are, you would like to move your life from where it is now to a far better place. Seeing how you've come this far, we should cover this very important aspect of recovery. Why? Because it will make a huge difference.

The influence of physical activity and its connection to depression is so often underestimated. We can confidently draw a parallel between the lack of physical activity in our TV and computer-dominated society and the alarming increase in mental and emotional-related illness in the western culture. I'm not saying that a physical exercise routine will solve everything and instantly cure depression. I am saying however, that it will help and without doubt accelerate the recovery program.

It is interesting to note the Black Dog Institute paper[9] on exercise and depression which states:

"In addition to being helpful for depression, there are numerous physical health benefits of regular exercise that are well-established by research. These benefits include prevention of numerous (including life-threatening) medical conditions such as heart disease, type 2 diabetes, osteoporosis, strokes and certain types of cancer. At a population level, physical inactivity is ranked just behind cigarette smoking as a major cause of ill health. Therefore, regular exercise as a treatment for depression has the added benefit of improving general health and preventing serious diseases."

I did some research recently with an expert on nutrition and mental wellness. Smoking is so detrimental to mental wellness and it upsets many forms of medication from antidepressants to antipsychotics that it is simply scary. If you're reading this and cigarettes are an issue for you, do everything you can to get off them. Seek some help if need be. If your natural reaction to that statement is: "You're not telling me what to do," my question would be then, "Isn't it time you got over that whole rebellion thing anyway?" It's far better to get all rebellious and defiant against the tobacco companies who for years have been stealing your livelihood, quality of life and nice breath and in the process have shortened your life and stolen you from your grandchildren. My advice is to run from tobacco as if your life depended on it -because it probably does.

If you have tight abs, the six-pack stomach, and bulging biceps and triceps, well done, but that's not me or my story. We have a group of push bike enthusiasts who every Sunday, park their SUVs, take their bikes off their specially designed bike racks and ride up the hill near our church building. It's a big hill! It's one of those very twisted country roads that lead to a lookout overlooking the city. Frankly the thought of riding up it makes

9 http://www.blackdoginstitute.org.au/docs/ExerciseandDepression.pdf

me think, 'why would you?' I can understand riding down it. I'm okay with that. (If the truth be known, I actually do ride up this hill quite often, and it's an amazing road with incredible coastal views, but my bike has a motor on it. It's the way bikes were meant to be!)

This section is about how a regular Joe like me found something that made a significant difference in my life.

I am making a few assumptions in this section. I'm assuming that my reader probably doesn't have a regular exercise routine. If you do, that's good and this section hopefully will encourage you to continue. Depression and mental-related problems can strike even the fittest and healthiest of us, however when I came to this significant aspect of recovery I was neither healthy nor fit.

I'm also assuming that my reader has perhaps tried and failed to remain active, and like me, you may top the scales higher then you should.

I'm a cake-eating, chocolate-loving, food fanatic. I love food! While reaching for the dessert, part of me is saying, "don't do it", and the other part (the one that usually wins) is saying, "Oh yeah, this will be good." It's like having shoulder angels who appear only when a dessert is near or I'm hanging out with the candies and chocolates in supermarkets.

This is me: I lick a postage stamp and put on weight. I've been known to put on a few pounds just chewing on a good idea. Some of my favorite movies are: Drop Dead Freddo, The Malteaser Falcon, The Curious Case of Benjamin Chocolate Buttons and Romper Chomper.

But there is hope.

I haven't become a marathon runner or buffed, muscular specimen of physical perfection. But what I did made a difference to me and I know you can do the same.

A bit of back story here will help. The story begins with Roger, who was a work associate and friend of mine. Roger took his son to New Zealand to walk the Milford Track. He had completed the walk many years before and had such a great experience that he decided to return. Roger and I had spoken about this walk and I really wanted to take Robyn. So I booked the flights, accommodation and dates for the trek.

Now, the Milford Track is a four-day trek with inspirational scenery in the beautiful Fiordland of New Zealand. But there was a problem: I was overweight, a chronic asthmatic and extremely unfit. Within the previous three years I had been housebound for extended periods with pneumonia twice and was also so run down that my hair fell out in clumps as alopecia left bald patches all over my head. But I booked it anyway.

My work was mentally draining but not physical at all. I knew I had to at least reach some sort of level of fitness and that meant training. Sorry for swearing! I had two previous attempts at gym work and both failed miserably. I still have emotional scarring from the 'pinch' test at the first gym I went to. The gym was not an option for me.

I needed to do something to get fitter, so I filled a backpack with heavy articles and walked around the suburbs of Campbelltown and Leumeah in Sydney's south west every chance I could. I must have looked quite a sight, with my borrowed military camouflage backpack and hiking boots, covered head to toe in perspiration as I walked the streets and bush land near my home in the middle of summer. I trained, we made it to Milford and completed the walk and it was one of the greatest experiences of my life.

I learnt something profound on this walk; it was almost an epiphany. I had imagined that while doing this walk, which was physically strenuous, I would be exhausted and fall into my bunk at night and sleep like a log.

However, this was not the case. I found that after walking with a very heavy pack uphill all day, I was buzzing—so much so that I hardly slept more than three hours each night. It was interesting to note as well that I ate not nearly as much food as I expected either. Back in Australia I worked long hours and finished exhausted by the end of the day without really any physical exercise. And I seemed to be always exhausted from mental stress.

I learned later that during that physical exercise of walking each day, I was producing a neurotransmitter called serotonin which is linked to mood, sleep, appetite and other functions. I felt more alive than I had felt for years while doing the very thing that should have exhausted me.

I felt great, and although at times during the walk I was exhausted physically, at the end of each day I was mentally buzzing, sharp as a tack and my thinking was clear as crystal. The fogginess that sometimes descends on our thinking was gone!

I knew in a few days I was heading back to Australia and into 'normal life'. How would I take this feeling back into my everyday world? I knew that if I didn't somehow begin to discipline myself upon my return, what I learnt would be lost.

I would love at this point to say, "I implemented an exercise routine from that day forward and now buy my latest exercise machine for three easy payments of $59.95."

I didn't, and in fact I failed many times to establish an exercise routine. Even though I now knew and had experienced the link between physical exercise and mental wellbeing I still struggled to do it! We generally know what we need to do, don't we?

Now, years later, I have an exercise routine. It's not flash or fancy. I don't get up every morning and start my day with a 20km bike ride, a 5km swim and 42km run. If you do—great! I still have days where everything in me does not want to go walking, even though I know I need to and I know how it helps me. The snooze button is still my nemesis. However, I now have an exercise routine and you can too!

Here is what I do. I walk! My body was not designed to run. I set the alarm and get up. (It's not as easy as it sounds!)

For you the right routine might be going to the gym or jogging, rowing or even surfing. The actual routine is not the real issue, it's getting into a routine that makes the difference.

Whatever option you take, it has to work for you. A friend of mine starts his day with a gym and bike routine with an instructor yelling at him. This works for him. It sounds like hell to me.

Another option to consider is having someone exercise with you. This can be great for motivation and accountability.

I get up and before I turn on the computer or the television or the coffee machine, I go walking. I know myself well enough to know that I'll get distracted as soon as they're on. I'll check emails and read something and send a reply and before you know it, I've missed my walk for that day. I've done this so many times. If the TV is on I'll watch the news and do the flick and then the children are up and the house is happening and I miss my walk for that day as well. It's so easy!

So I get up before the family, get into my walking gear, drink a glass of water, eat nothing and head off. The first five minutes can be agony but mostly now it's just great to get on my walk. Once I get into it I enjoy it. It takes me 45 minutes to go down our bush driveway, turn left and travel along the road till its end. Then I touch the pole on the corner, turn around and head back home through a rural housing estate. It's 45 minutes of doing a decent pace, enough to work up a sweat. This is not 'power walking' or doing that hip thing those Olympic walkers do. I simply walk at a consistent pace and I do this four to five days a week and I have found it transformational in my life. It will be transformational in your life as well.

I like going early because it starts my day on the right foot, or path, or track, depending on the pun I'd like to use. It clears my head and without doubt helps me think clearer throughout the rest of the day.

I tried all sorts of things like reading before I headed off and meditating on what I read as I walked. That's cool and worth trying but it didn't really work for me. This is probably because I tend to get distracted easily.

I've found that to head off on my walk even while half asleep (although in winter I tend to wake up pretty quickly) is the best way for me to start my day.

I think, I pray and I meditate but sometimes I just simply walk and I'm sure I've hardly thought about anything the whole time.

If you're a thinker and your brain runs a million miles an hour like mine—commit to thinking positively while walking! It's too easy to think negatively so you have to purposefully think about something positive.

There is a passage from the Bible I have found helpful in this process.

Philippians 4:8

Finally, whatever is true, whatever is noble, whatever is right, whatever is pure, whatever is lovely, whatever is admirable—if anything is excellent or praiseworthy—think about such things.

When I start to think negatively about someone or something, I stop myself and find something good to think about. Even if it's the fact that I got off my lazy butt, defeated the evil snooze button and went for a walk, that's a positive!

SO HOW TO GET STARTED

Generally speaking it takes about 30 days to create a good habit and if you're like me, about 30 seconds to create a bad one. So what we are trying to do is create a good habit.

We need to set realistic goals. For anyone who has not exercised for a long time and sets out saying, "Okay, I will now walk for 45 minutes every day for the next 30 days," their chances of success are next to zero! For a start, if you're not used to walking and you start with 45 minutes of vigorous walking, it will probably half-kill you. You will feel it the next day and the day after and you will find it very hard to do again. One of the biggest problems for anyone who starts an exercise routine, be it gym work, running or any other type of program, is that they go too hard to fast and don't last!

So, my recommendation is this: start with a shorter time and aim for three to four days a week. Start with 15 minutes, three days a week, than increase to half an hour and work your way to 45 minutes and four to five days a week. Remember, you are implementing something that on paper looks easy, yet in practice is difficult. Your body will not thank you for this at the beginning! It will most likely fight you every step (pardon the pun again) of the way. But we are talking about your mental, emotional and physical health, your life expectancy, your quality of life, your relationships and even your wealth. Every aspect of your life will be affected positively by doing this. You can do this! If a cake-eating, sweets-loving, chocoholic like me can, so can you!

STUBBORN DETERMINATION

Prepare yourself: you watch, as soon as you get out there and start, some super fit 'muscles on muscles' person will jog past you without breaking a sweat. The lycra-clad peloton will ride by all looking fit with their skin-tight outfits and calf muscles the size of grapefruits bulging on each leg. The lady with the midriff exercise top showing off her tight six-pack stomach will smile as she glides past, making it all seem so easy.

Expect it! It will happen. Expect it, but ignore it as well. Don't ignore them—they may look superhuman but in reality they're just people—but ignore the feelings of inadequacy you will have about yourself and just keep going. Wear dark sunglasses and a hat if you have to! Remember, this is about your health not theirs.

Ask yourself, "How silly it would be if I let others stop me from becoming well?"

Be prepared that everything will try and stop you doing this. Your body will hate you, for a while. Actually this changes after a while, as once you have established the habit your body will thank you and even miss the routine when it's interrupted. Things will happen to disrupt your routine. The weather! We now live near Coffs Harbour on the stunning North Coast of New South Wales, Australia. Around our area we have very high rain fall. It rains a lot! When it rains here it's 'gully washer' stuff. This is another reason why I don't say I will do my 45 minutes every day, because I won't, and if it's pouring rain I'm not going out to catch pneumonia. In this case, or if you live in a predominantly cold or hot climate, having a treadmill inside is a good idea.

It will take determination, and the more determined you need to be, the greater the sense of achievement will be. I want you to be selfish in regards to this. Why? Because I know this; you will be far better in every aspect of your life and for others if you do. So, by being selfish and getting an exercise routine established, you are actually doing the most unselfish thing you can do. That's pretty cool!

It will take determination to get the habit created and a decision that says, "All right, I'm doing this no matter what. No further correspondence will be entered into."

I've been doing this for years now and I love it but even after a break if I'm sick or traveling for a week or it's been like this last week in Coffs Harbour—extremely wet—that first walk can be difficult. So it will take determination, however great benefits are obtained by gritting your teeth and persisting.

For the next 30 days create a good habit in your life and see the difference. If I can, anyone can!

DIET

Dietary advice must always be considered in the light of your personal health status. If you have a medical condition that requires you eat certain foods at certain times, for example diabetes, then you will know if you must obey any medical requirements. Any suggestions I make must be considered in the light of your personal medical status and advice.

After my walk, and even on the days I don't walk, I eat a healthy breakfast. Make your breakfast full of food that gets your system functioning. This book is not a cook book, and there is plenty of good material about what is healthy and what's not healthy to eat.

There is an old saying that goes: we are what we eat. That doesn't mean I turn into a hot dog if I eat one. However, consistent change over time produces results.

I read once this statement: "Right things done repeatedly produce right results." This is so true, however the reverse is true as well. Wrong things done repeatedly produce wrong results. For instance: if I eat a chocolate bar once today, it will make very little difference. However, if I were to eat a chocolate bar every day for the next year, I would start to notice an effect, wouldn't I? (I'm still working out whether that illustration fits into the positive or negative. I love my chocolate!)

Here are a few things I've dropped out of my diet that over time have made a huge difference: Sugary fizzy drinks, high sugar breakfast cereals, potato chips, fast food burgers and fries, ice-cream and biscuits. I also reduced my intake of breads, and I love fresh bread. I could eat a bakery full of fresh bread. I also discovered that my body has an adverse reaction to MSG, otherwise known in Australia as flavor enhancer 621.

The reason I removed these items is very simple. They are weight gain and early death in fancy wrappings. For an example, let's use sugary fizzy drinks. Sugar needs to be burnt up or it turns to fat and results in weight gain. It took me a long time to realize that those slim, bikini-clad, beautiful models that advertise certain fizzy drinks would probably never drink the stuff, or very little of it if they did, otherwise they would not be slim nor look that great in bikinis. Even with diet fizzy drinks there is enough evidence to show how bad these are for our bodies. Here is a news flash: we don't actually need them and the great thing is we have a choice. We don't have to drink them! Remember, this is cake-loving, sweets-eating, chocoholic Gary speaking. I'm not asking you to become a vegetarian or vegan overnight. Your body will go into shock if you do. Have you ever tried to go cold turkey off caffeine? Your head feels like it's about to explode!

Balance is the issue here. Make changes and stick to them and the results will come! Making the right choices repeatedly brings the right results.

CHILL A BIT

Sorry to break it to you, but you will more than likely mess up some times. When you do, don't throw in the towel and say, "it's all too hard, I can never change". You can change and you can recover and you can implement and sustain an exercise routine in your life. One of the greatest lessons I have learnt is to forgive myself and to say: "OK, I messed up, and probably really enjoyed messing up. That ice cream sundae was amazing."

Start again. Do a John Wayne and get back on your horse.

The world is full of people who just give up. You're here today reading this book because something inside you does not want to give up. Or perhaps you did give up but today you're making a choice not to any longer. Something deep inside is crying out for change and we know no change is easy. Just forgive yourself and start again. I remember a very wise man said to me once: "Do you know the great thing about yesterday? It finished at midnight." Today is a new day and it's also the first day of the rest of our lives.

DISCIPLINE IS THE KEY

You might remember when we looked at the biblical passage that describes God giving us a spirit of 'love, power and a sound mind', we revealed that the 'sound mind' referred not to some heavenly zap to fix all, but to 'obtaining a sound mind through self discipline'. The self discipline of creating an exercise routine in our lives is an essential ingredient in obtaining this sound mind that God gives.

A friend of mine years ago coined a phrase that certainly lived long in the memory of our children and still, over a decade later, comes up in conversation. He used to say: "Don't say I can't, say how can I?" Take those same words of wisdom into this process today. Don't say I can't, say how can I?

When you try and fail, don't say I can't, say how can I?

When those bikini-clad beauties make you feel inadequate, don't quit! Don't say I can't, say how can I?

When the burgers and fries are calling, when the fizzy, high-sugar drinks demand attention, when the snooze button seeks to steal your achievements, or when the perfect peloton peddle past in procession, then let everything within rise up in destiny-defining determination and scream it from every fiber of your being. "Don't say I can't, say how can I?"

Then go again, and again, and again, and again till there is a routine in your life. When you have it, keep it.

From a sweets-loving, chocoholic to you: if I can, so can you.

"DE-VUE-IST-SPECTAC-LAR"

STEP 6: THE MUST OF TRUST

"I cannot take another step," Robyn exclaimed as she sat down on a rock, "It's so high and I'm so tired." I was struggling also, but being male, didn't let on as much. It was our second day walking the Milford Track, in the stunningly beautiful Fiordland National Park, New Zealand. For years I had wanted to do this four-day walk and this was our first step into the realm of being trekkers.

But it had not been an easy day. We did this trek the 'real' way. There was none of this champagne-style stuff, staying in flash accommodation with hot showers and restaurant prepared meals. Not for us! It was full packs and no showers, cook your own food sort of style. Our packs were also very heavy. As we walked through these glacier-cut valleys beside rivers fed from melting snow, we were in awe of this amazing area but it had been 18 kilometers of constant uphill grade before we finished at the foot of the mountain pass. Did I mention that we were carrying huge heavy packs?

A few weeks before flying to New Zealand to start the walk, a friend of mine in Australia who had done it, said that if the weather was fine on day two we should try to get to the top of the pass and see the view. The weather in New Zealand, and especially the southern mountain regions, can change incredibly quickly. The weather that day was perfect, so Robyn and I decided to go up the pass, so as not to miss the opportunity of seeing what very few ever get to see. We were also inspired in a different way by a man we met just before we started who said rather negatively, "Good luck! I've done the walk three times and have never seen the view from the top." Not to let a chance go by, we set off.

This was a huge challenge for us but we set off, me with my asthma, and Robyn with a strong fear of heights. The climb was steep and it zigzagged back and forth across the mountain face as we climbed higher and higher. In one place, a part of the track had been taken out by a land slide and we had to climb up a rope to reach the next zig (or zag). We were completely exhausted. To even attempt this thing was huge for us both. As we climbed higher, and reached above the tree line, it became quite exposed. Robyn's fear of heights kicked in. It became very difficult for us both. So on the rock we sat, head in hands, tired, fearful (Robyn, not me) and physically exhausted. We had zigged and zagged our way up a long distance but we were done. We could not stay there so we had a choice before us; keep on going up, or turn back. It was right then that one of these 'true trekkers', the kind who can climb anything and not ever break out in a sweat, came past us on his way down. He had been to the top and as he went past us, sitting there quite dejected, he simply said, "Not dat fa to go, nd de-vue-ist-spectaclar." We translated it to; "there's not that far to go, and the view is spectacular." It was enough for Robyn and me to lift ourselves up and keep stepping forward. That last part of the trek, however long it was, was just plain hard work, but when we took those last steps onto the high mountain pass, the beauty of what unfolded before us took our breath away. (Actually, I was pretty well out of breath anyway, but it was stunning). We found ourselves standing in what must be one of the most beautiful places on earth. The mountains and valleys stretched out before us. This 360-degree view was the most stunning thing I had ever seen.

To this day, I can still see it, with all the splendor of creation laid out before us. We were on top of the world. The exhaustion, effort and pain seemed suddenly worth every step. When I think of what we would have missed if we had turned back when things were difficult, and how close we were to doing just that, it sets me wondering. How many times do we turn back just before we are about to accomplish something wonderful? How many times are we so close to the breakthrough in our lives we so desire, yet turn back when it gets difficult? Today, if you're sitting on a rock and thinking you cannot go any further; it's too hard, the road is too steep; if you're full of fear because you have never been to these heights before or you're not too sure how far the zigzags keep going on or you're even feeling exposed to the elements, let me be the friend who walks past you, just like 'Mr Trekker' did for us those years ago.

Although I cannot put on his thick European accent, I can say to you today, "Keep going, it's not as far as you may think, just keep your eyes on going forward and not returning or going back down the mountain. Take the next step and the one after, one step at a time. The view truly is spectacular—the clearness of the air, and the beauty of God's creation open around us. You can do this thing."

When we've come so far, we need to seize our moments. By the way, the next day when we climbed the pass again it was foggy and we could see virtually nothing. I'm so glad we kept climbing and that we were able to see that amazing view.

I'm also glad I took the step forward that we are about to discuss in the process of reaching above depression and mental illness. This step will help us see beyond our limitations and into the spectacular. This step is what I call 'choosing to trust God, more than trusting what I think'.

This is not as easy as it sounds, and if you're like me, I tend to try to figure everything out. I sort it all out in my mind and then advise God on what action He should take. It may just be me, but if you're quietly chuckling to yourself and nodding, it might just be you as well! I'm still waiting for that very special day when the God of all creation will appear in a heavenly vision before me with a host of heavenly beings with trumpets, robes, wings and an abundance of haloes, and say something like, "Wow, thanks Gary, I hadn't thought of that. I'm implementing a coordinated strategy plan around your suggestion immediately. Thank you so much, Gary. You're a legend. I honestly don't know how I could run this whole God's kingdom thing without you." I think you would agree there is very little chance of that ever happening. Actually, there is no chance! It's funny to imagine this scenario or to think of God reacting that way. Yet when I look at my life I wonder how many times do I actually think I've got a better handle on the situation than God, or understand all the complex variables in a given situation than God. I have a nagging suspicion that many of us so often tend to do this very thing.

This is how it plays out some times; it's what I think first, and if what God says fits into that, well and good. The challenge comes when what I think is different to what God says.

There's a small verse in Psalm 119 that says something interesting;

Psalm 119:59

I thought about my ways, and turned my feet to your testimonies.

Our thoughts will always go to our ways, but it's how we choose to walk that makes all the difference. This verse says "I turned my feet", so I turned my choice and my actions to God's ways. Very simply; I choose to take God's word over what I think.

I'm not necessarily talking about some of the easy to identify choices. For instance, if I think I would like to kill someone, God's word says, 'You should not kill.' That's an easy one—well, it should be. Mind you, I have met some people that have really tempted me on this!

What about a married man having sex with another woman? 'You should not commit adultery.' The list goes on, and these are fundamentals of the Christian life. Another would be having sexual relations outside of the purity of marriage. Clearly God talks about fornication and about purity in the scriptures. These are clear and generally understood. Thankfully God's nature is mercy and grace. Just remember this before we move on. Available to us, no matter what circumstances we find ourselves in, is God's grace.

In Deuteronomy, God is talking to people who have wandered a long way from God's optimum plan for their lives yet He says this;

Deuteronomy 4:29 (MSG)

But even there, if you seek God, your God, you'll be able to find him if you're serious, looking for him with your whole heart and soul.

This grace is given freely by the hand of a loving heavenly Father. You may find yourself in a situation where bad choices, or even good choices that have gone bad, have led you to a place where things seem wrong in every way. God's mercies are new every morning, the Bible says. It's where we go from here that will count. All journeys have a start and finish. Lots of us have to start and restart many times along that journey. Let us all be those who determine to finish well. No one remembers how a person starts a race, but it's how they finish that counts.

Remember that from where you are, God can build something beautiful if you let him. God is all about building a brighter future and a better tomorrow. We are where we are right now because of the choices we have made leading to this point. When it comes to trusting God more than our own thoughts, we need to believe that God can, and desires to, make the best of any situation we find ourselves in.

BELIEVING IN GOD, OR BELIEVING GOD?

When it comes to taking God at His word rather than what we think, we must ask ourselves a question. Do I believe *in* God, or believe God? The correct answer would be both 'I believe *in* God, and I believe God'. That little word 'in' is huge here. There is a massive difference between these. We can believe in God for salvation and forgiveness. We can easily believe in His love and reality, and so we should.

It is easy to believe *in* God, but when it comes to simply believing God, or taking Him at His word, we can come unstuck.

The belief in God can take on many forms. "There is a supreme being in the cosmos, I know there must be. I just don't know what or who it is," or, "I go to church each Sunday and I believe in God," or, "I don't go to any fellowship or church but I'm a believer, I love Jesus," and so on.

Let's give this a practical application. What about the young, stirred-up, genuine Christ-following woman who hits 30 and has no husband, and who looks around her church group but without seeing any real possibilities on the horizon? As time goes by, a friend from work invites her to a dinner party. At the dinner party is a young man and they start talking. He's a nice enough person and he asks her out on a date. He's not a Christ-follower but he's a nice person. He treats her well and may even be a gentleman at heart. She has told him that sex outside marriage is not happening because of her faith, and he's okay with that.

As time goes by they become good friends, and she feels a sense of security when he's around. That fear of being alone doesn't nag her yet she knows she is faced with a choice. The Bible clearly says not to be unequally yoked with a non-believer. This is easy to say if you're not alone, in your 30s or possibly a young single mum. What if these two people are a match in every way except in their belief in God?

Here is the point: in these types of situations we have a

choice. Will I be a believer *in* God or will I really believe God and take His word as the ultimate authority for my life? Will I choose to stand on what I think? The thought in this situation may be, "Perhaps I can lead him to Christ," or, "Given time, he will come to Christ by my example." But what you're actually saying is, "Did God really say you shouldn't be unequally yoked to an unbeliever?"

Surely God wants you to be happy. He's a God of love and He will understand. This is a very challenging situation that many find themselves in. I do not want to be insensitive about this, as the thought of spending life alone is frightening for so many of us. And I know we could get all supposedly spiritual and say, "We are not really alone when we have Christ," and this is true. However, it really doesn't help so many in this situation. I have seen beautiful young women throw away their future and God's great plan for their lives by running after someone who may be a nice person. But to go that way is to go against God's word. These are the points of decision that alter our lives. Some would say destiny lies in these moments. God has a plan for each and every life on this planet, and His plan is far greater and larger than our human minds can fathom. His thoughts are so much greater than our thoughts. I think it's a good time to remind ourselves of one of the most quoted scripture passages in the world today.

Jeremiah 29:11

"For I know the plans I have for you," declares the LORD, "plans to prosper you and not to harm you, plans to give you hope and a future."

The Message Bible puts it this way:

"I know what I'm doing. I have it all planned out—plans to take care of you, not abandon you, plans to give you the future you hope for."

GOD'S OPTIMUM PLAN

God has an optimum plan for our lives, and I believe that even if we may have missed that optimum plan years ago, He has an optimum plan from this point on until the completion of our lives.

What if we, by rushing into a situation that is not the optimum plan of God, actually throw away or miss the greatest plan of all? If we see God for who He is in His boundless love for each one of us, it strengthens our trust. His desire is for the best for all for us. Not only is it His desire, but He acts upon His plans. Let's not settle for second best. Someone once said, "God takes full responsibility for those whose hearts are fully His."

The above scenario and many others like it are the things that challenge us in life. Our heart and our thoughts want to go one way but God's word says something different. It's when your heart wants to run and God says 'stay' that we choose to either be a believer *in* God, or to believe God.

Another scenario could be when the husband is having trouble at work and home is full of difficulty. The children may be suffering with illness, and his once-beautiful wife is aging, struggling with shattered self-esteem and troubles at home. He arrives home from work and the house is not the perfect place it was when it was just the two of them. The meal is perhaps not up to the standard he desires, and the children are so noisy that he cannot hear the television. The beautiful young woman he married, still the love of his life, is struggling with her weight, and her nice clothes are too often replaced with less glamorous cheap tracksuit pants.

It's a difficult time in their lives. Christmas is coming up, and the office has its party planned. His wife cannot go, because one of the children has a disorder that means someone needs to be with them at all times. So he goes to the party alone. There he meets a female colleague who has just come through a divorce and is still very lonely and sad. Yet this time, something is there that has not been there before. She compliments him on his clothes and how he looks because he's lost a bit of weight. He feels good about himself for what seems to be the first time for ages. They don't go running off to the nearest motel and sleep together, in fact the thought has not even entered his mind. He's a godly, church-attending man who loves his wife and family. Things are difficult at the moment, but he's committed to his family. Time goes by, and the friendship at work becomes closer. She confides in him about her difficulty, and he also confides in her about other things. No physical contact takes place until one day after a lunch together where they talk about their difficulties, she thanks him for his caring words and kisses his cheek. It's nothing really, yet he knows she likes and appreciates him, and he genuinely likes her friendship and listening ear as well. He also realizes that contained in that small, seemingly insignificant kiss on the cheek is a possible something more.

Here again is the choice. He knows that it may not be today, it may not be tomorrow, but sooner or later, the time will come when he will have an opportunity to start again in life. He will be able to walk away from all the troubles at home and start a new life with a new woman who obviously loves and appreciates him. He does not really want to. He loves his children and wife. The Bible clearly talks about adultery and about how sacred the marriage relationship is. So what does he do? Does he end up leaving his wife or have an affair, still being a believer *in* God, or does he stand on what God says about the relationship in the marriage? Will I be a believer *in* God and do what *I* think is best for me, or will I stand on His word and believe God, trusting that through the difficulties, our relationships can become even better?

I know the above-mentioned hypothetical examples are a little bit 'Mills and Boon-ish'. I also don't want to be insensitive to anyone who has gone through similar situations, and who perhaps has been faced with these very real choices. However,

I hope they illustrate graphically that we can still be believers *in* God, yet live lives that show that we don't really believe God. If the truth be known, we have all in varying degrees been believers *in* God and not believed God. This is not to point a finger at anyone. If it were, I would have to point the finger at myself more than anyone else. This section is to encourage us all to believe God, meaning, simply to put the authority of God's written word above all our thoughts and ideas.

To look at a biblical example, the difference between King Saul and King David shows how it works. Let us go to probably the most familiar passage in the Bible, the classic true story of David and Goliath. This story has been preached about millions of times. Sunday schools have taught it constantly. We even joke about it as Sunday school teachers, saying, "What will we do this Sunday? I know, let's do David and Goliath." Apart from the death and resurrection of Christ, David and Goliath would probably be the most taught passage of scripture in the world. Now there is nothing wrong with that. It is a great story of good conquering evil. The little guy beats the big, mean, ugly, smelly, nasty giant. You've got to love a good underdog story! Particularly the part where this young man calls out to the big, ugly giant, "I'm going to cut your big, fat head off", when he doesn't even have a sword to do it with.

I'm not going to blow your minds with some amazing revelation that no one has ever seen before in this passage. However, the reason I point it out is because it shows clearly that we can be believers in God, and still not believe God, whatever our circumstances.

BELIEVING IN, YET NOT BELIEVING

I will tell the story, and then include some verses. However I encourage you to read all of 1 Samuel chapter 17. Two armies were lined up in battle formation; the Philistines and their arch enemies, the Israelites. The Israelites were, at that time and throughout the Old Testament, referred to as the children of God. We can say today that the Israelite army were believers *in* God. You could have asked any of them, and they would have said they were God's people and they believed *in* Him. They knew their history and how God had done great things for them. They worshipped at the temple. They had traditions of godliness throughout their culture and lives. They were led by a king who was a believer *in* God. He did all the right things to show his belief in God. Yet when he and his army saw big, huge Goliath of Gath come forward to fight them, they ran for cover because these believers *in* God simply didn't believe God. They had come through great victories and there were strong and mighty men in their number. These were not a pack of spineless wimps who couldn't fight their way out of a wet paper bag. These men were strong soldiers who had seen action before and won great victories. Yet at this time, in these circumstances, this army of believers *in* God simply did not believe God. They saw the giant, and could not see that God was bigger.

Here is the choice again. Do we believe God? Or, do we let our actions show that we think that this circumstance we are in is far too big for God? What giants are you facing today?

Now your giant may be big. I would be the first to say that if your giant is named depression or mental illness, it's not just big, it's huge. Notice that David never denied the bigness of Goliath. This is a secret: Victory does not come in denying the bigness of an issue, it comes in the acknowledgment that God is bigger.

Remember, courage is only available when fear is present. Or, as it has been said, "Courage is not the absence of fear, but it comes in the choice that something is greater than that fear."

Let's read a bit together. We pick up the story when David is heading out to face Goliath on the battlefield.

1 Samuel 17:40-50

Then he took his staff in his hand, chose five smooth

stones from the stream, put them in the pouch of his shepherd's bag and, with his sling in his hand, approached the Philistine.

Meanwhile, the Philistine, with his shield bearer in front of him, kept coming closer to David. He looked David over and saw that he was only a boy, ruddy and handsome, and he despised him. He said to David, 'Am I a dog that you come at me with sticks?' And the Philistine cursed David by his gods. 'Come here', he said, 'and I'll give your flesh to the birds of the air and the beasts of the field!'

David said to the Philistine, 'You come against me with sword and spear and javelin, but I come against you in the name of the LORD Almighty, the God of the armies of Israel, whom you have defied. This day the LORD will hand you over to me, and I'll strike you down and cut off your head. Today I will give the carcasses of the Philistine army to the birds of the air and the beasts of the earth, and the whole world will know that there is a God in Israel. All those gathered here will know that it is not by sword or spear that the LORD saves; for the battle is the LORD's, and he will give all of you into our hands.'

As the Philistine moved closer to attack him, David ran quickly toward the battle line to meet him. Reaching into his bag and taking out a stone, he slung it and struck the Philistine on the forehead. The stone sank into his forehead, and he fell face down on the ground.

So David triumphed over the Philistine with a sling and a stone; without a sword in his hand he struck down the Philistine and killed him.

What made the difference?

Was it that David was a great shot with the sling and stone? It helped, but that's not it. David did not deny the size of Goliath.

Instead, he chose to acknowledge the size of God. That, my friend, is faith. Simply choosing to believe God, rather than just believing in God. Seeing the circumstance or situation, and choosing to take God at His word.

THE DEVIL IS IN THE DOUBT!

Right back in the very beginning, in the Garden of Eden, we see the example of how forces work in the heavenly realm. After Adam and Eve were created, God had given Adam instructions about the trees to eat from and the trees not to eat from. And then the evil one entered the scene. The devil has always been crafty and deceitful. His greatest weapon back then, as it is now, is to create doubt in our hearts that what God actually says is true. God had said this:

Genesis 2:15-17

The LORD God took the man and put him in the Garden of Eden to work it and take care of it. And the LORD God commanded the man, "You are free to eat from any tree in the garden; but you must not eat from the tree of the knowledge of good and evil, for when you eat of it you will surely die".

Look at how it plays out and we see that our evil enemy uses doubt to take control.

Genesis 3:1-11

Now the serpent was craftier than any of the wild animals the LORD God had made. He said to the woman, 'Did God really say, "You must not eat from any tree in the garden?"'

The woman said to the serpent, 'We may eat fruit from the trees in the garden, but God did say, "You must not eat fruit from the tree that is in the middle of the garden, and you must not touch it, or you will die".

'You will not surely die', the serpent said to the woman. 'For God knows that when you eat of it your eyes will be opened, and you will be like God, knowing good and evil.'

When the woman saw that the fruit of the tree was good for food and pleasing to the eye, and also desirable for gaining wisdom, she took some and ate it. She also gave some to her husband, who was with her, and he ate it. Then the eyes of both of them were opened, and they realized they were naked; so they sewed fig leaves together and made coverings for themselves.

Then the man and his wife heard the sound of the LORD God as he was walking in the garden in the cool of the day, and they hid from the LORD God among the trees of the garden. But the LORD God called to the man, "Where are you?"

He answered, 'I heard you in the garden, and I was afraid because I was naked; so I hid.'

And he said, "Who told you that you were naked? Have you eaten from the tree that I commanded you not to eat from?"

This phrase, '*did God really say?*' produced doubt and opened them up to suggestions, and eventually the fall of mankind.

It may be the ultimate oxymoron within Christianity to say that someone is a 'doubting believer'. I've doubted God many times and I still do sometimes. I challenge anyone who has been a believer for any length of time to tell the truth and confess the same. Let's be real. We all have situations arise, and they may be huge or small, where we are challenged to just be a believer *in* God, let alone actually believe God. Be encouraged to believe God today. That is to take 'His Word' over our thoughts and ideas.

CAN YOU WALK ON WATER?

Look at another classic Bible story with me for a moment. Peter walking on water is another one of those told-a-million-times passages. It is rich with imagery of a mortal man doing the impossible but succumbing to his human side in sinking, only to be rescued by Jesus' outstretched hand.

Matthew 14:22-33

Immediately Jesus made the disciples get into the boat and go on ahead of him to the other side, while he dismissed the crowd. After he had dismissed them, he went up on a mountainside by himself to pray. When evening came, he was there alone, but the boat was already a considerable distance from land, buffeted by the waves because the wind was against it.

During the fourth watch of the night Jesus went out to them, walking on the lake. When the disciples saw him walking on the lake, they were terrified. 'It's a ghost', they said, and cried out in fear.

But Jesus immediately said to them: "Take courage! It is I. Don't be afraid."

'Lord, if it's you,' Peter replied, 'tell me to come to you on the water.'

'Come,' he said.

Then Peter got down out of the boat, walked on the water and came toward Jesus. But when he saw the wind, he was afraid and, beginning to sink, cried out, 'Lord, save me!'

Immediately Jesus reached out his hand and caught him. "You of little faith," he said, "why did you doubt?"

And when they climbed into the boat, the wind died down. Then those who were in the boat worshiped him, saying, 'Truly you are the Son of God.'

Just think about this for a moment. What was Peter actually walking on? What do you think? Water! Look at it this way. You or I could say, "Okay, I'm a believer. So anything that Peter did, I can do too." We could stir ourselves up and set off to the beach and start to walk. Try it if you want—but take a towel. If there is no beach or ocean around, a lake is fine. Just don't be surprised when you get wet. Classic Pentecostalism would say something like, "Well you didn't have the faith." Perhaps, but that is not the reason, and having the faith was not the reason that Peter was able to walk on water, even for the time he did. Yes it requires faith to believe God—or is it in believing God that faith is born? Remember all the other disciples believed *in* God, yet Peter was the one who believed God, stepped out, and walked on the command of Christ. The water was certainly there, but Peter was walking on what Jesus said, and the promise contained *within* the command. He was walking on the Word of God. He simply took Jesus at His word, '*come*'.

The word Jesus said was '*come*' and this simple word had incredible power because it was God's instruction to Peter at that time. The instruction was not to produce some hyper-faith reaction that says today, "I'll walk on water, you just watch me." God has not instructed us to walk on water. Metaphorically, the things that God has instructed us to walk on are His words found within the scriptures. These words are what we are able to walk through life on. The wind and the waves of our lives will come, however we are able, by the command of God, to walk through any and all situations.

The word 'tell' in verse 28 (or in the King James Version 'bid'), is the Greek word *keleuo*, meaning 'to command or order'. Peter was not moving from that boat without the command of God, because, as impulsive as Peter was, he knew that the command of God was stronger than his faith, and *within* God's commands, the miraculous can be achieved. We know that Peter started walking on water (and as far as I am aware, he is still the only one apart from Jesus who has actually done that). But Peter started to look around him and began to think, and doubt crept in. The Bible says that he '*saw the wind*', when actually you cannot see wind. Really, he saw the evidence of the strength of the wind. He saw the waves, and his focus left God's command of '*come*', and turned to his circumstances. I think we can safely say that Peter was a believer and a Christ-follower, and that he meant well. He still believed *in* God, yet his eyes were distracted and his focus on believing God's command and walking on that was destroyed by doubt. When his eyes were turned from Jesus and His command, he started to get that sinking feeling—pardon the pun. Jesus rescued him and asked him, "Why did you doubt?"

It's not in the easy stuff of life that we doubt God generally. It's when challenges come. It's when things are not clear. It's when the wind and waves of life crash around us. Yet it's in those times that if we just hold to God's word (His command) and obey, simply believing God, that we are strengthened through all life's circumstances. Doubt will overpower the voice of God in our lives every time.

In Ephesians Chapter 6, it talks about the armor of God and lists the equipment we need to stand strong in God. Here is a question for you: has the devil penetrated through your defenses with the 'doubting dart'?

Ephesians 6:16-17

In addition to all this, take up the shield of faith, with which you can extinguish all the flaming arrows of the evil one. Take the helmet of salvation and the sword of the Spirit, which is the word of God.

A SLICE OF SUPREME

Our thoughts will bring about doubt as we get caught up in the circumstances of life. It is only by God's Word that we can stand to overcome. To believe God, we must place what He says as the supreme authority for our lives. This is vital to progress and imperative to reach life beyond depression and mental illness.

Is my giant big? Yes. But God is, believe it or not, bigger!

THINKING THIS THROUGH

Let us take a look at how God describes the brilliance of our thinking compared to His. Are you ready? It hurts by the way! Say "ouch" with me before we start.

Psalm 94:11

The LORD knows the thoughts of man; he knows that they are futile.

Ouch!

Futile! That's very encouraging God, thanks for that! But when we really think about this, it is true. All our plotting and planning is futile compared to God's unlimited understanding. Combine that with His endless love and compassion for us, and we see a combination far more trustworthy than our own thoughts.

Psalm 94:11 (KJV)

The LORD knoweth the thoughts of man, that they are vanity.

The word 'vanity', from the Hebrew word *habel,* describes something that is completely futile and that comes up so short that it is like an empty breath that vanishes in a moment.

The King James Version calls it 'vanity' when we try and out-think God. We're out of line and we will mess it up. I have learned that the eternal truths found in the scriptures lead to life and happiness, while my way of thinking generally only leads me to sadness and emptiness. The Bible simply states it this way: *'know the truth and the truth will set you free.'* **John 8:32**

Not just having the truth but knowing and applying the truth is the key to this statement. I have personally found this to be true! I have learnt that God knows me better than I know myself;

Psalm 139:1-3

O LORD, you have searched me and you know me.

You know when I sit and when I rise; you perceive my thoughts from afar.

You discern my going out and my lying down; you are familiar with all my ways.

He is also trustworthy to help me. He is after all, '*Our help in a time of need.*' **Hebrews 4:16** I can cast my burden upon Him because He cares for me.

Isaiah 55:8-9

"For my thoughts are not your thoughts, neither are your ways my ways." declares the LORD.

"As the heavens are higher than the earth, so are my ways higher than your ways, and my thoughts than your thoughts."

What about when it comes to issues in our lives? Will we take God's Word, or our thinking into issues of life? God's ways are so much higher than our ways, and His understanding goes far beyond our understanding. He sees the whole picture while, we see only the back of the tapestry.

I have learned that God has better plans for me—better than I could ever have for myself.

WORSHIP

Most people wait until they feel a certain way before acting upon things. Many people with depression, emotional instability and mental illness avoid worship and cut themselves off from worship services because they don't feel like they are worthy to be there or to sing praises to God. Yet this is contrary to what God says. He tells us not to forsake gathering together, and to worship corporately. So what do I choose? My thoughts or God's word? Will I proclaim being a believer *in* God yet not believe Him? The real trick in this is to act before we feel. The feelings will follow the act of obedience to what God says.

Worship is important to me because I believe it is a great weapon in the war for our minds. There is an indescribable, incredible power in praising our God. The Bible tells us to come before God with *'shouts of praise, loudly worshipping and singing to our God'*, **Psalm 95:1-2** using our emotions to worship. The Bible tells us to, *'put on the garment of praise for the spirit of heaviness.'* **Isaiah 61:3 (NKJV)**

2 Chronicles 20 tells a story of how powerful praising God is in the fight against insurmountable odds. I believe depression and mental illness can be a fight against insurmountable odds. So what can we do practically?

In this chapter of the bible, we see an impossible situation facing people who were believers in God. A vast army was coming against them to destroy every trace of God's people. King Jehoshaphat was alarmed, and he took the situation to God. The battle plan God gave them was, to the natural way of thinking, rather stupid, but then again we don't wage war as the world does. Our weapons are mighty to pull down strongholds by the power of God. Our greatest weapon is to be obedient to what God says.

2 Chronicles 20:16-22

"Tomorrow march down against them. They will be climbing up by the Pass of Ziz, and you will find them at the end of the gorge in the Desert of Jeruel. You will not have to fight this battle. Take up your positions; stand firm and see the deliverance the LORD will give you, O Judah

and Jerusalem. Do not be afraid; do not be discouraged. Go out to face them tomorrow, and the LORD will be with you."

Jehoshaphat bowed with his face to the ground, and all the people of Judah and Jerusalem fell down in worship before the LORD. Then some Levites from the Kohathites and Korahites stood up and praised the LORD, the God of Israel, with very loud voice.

Early in the morning they left for the Desert of Tekoa. As they set out, Jehoshaphat stood and said, 'Listen to me, Judah and people of Jerusalem! Have faith in the LORD your God and you will be upheld; have faith in his prophets and you will be successful.' After consulting the people, Jehoshaphat appointed men to sing to the LORD and to praise him for the splendour of his holiness as they went out at the head of the army, saying: 'Give thanks to the LORD, for his love endures forever.'

As they began to sing and praise, the LORD set ambushes against the men of Ammon and Moab and Mount Seir who were invading Judah, and they were defeated.

Just think about this for a moment. God told them to leave the only protection they had in the natural sense, and head out against a huge enemy. Not only that, they were to sing and praise their God while they were doing it. So before any of their enemies had been defeated, they had to choose to trust what God said over what they thought. They could not stay in their hiding places being just believers *in* God, so they stepped out and sang, believing God and taking Him at His word, and a great victory was won.

If you know, or have known Christ and you have not worshipped Him for a while, start again now! No matter how you feel, do it anyway. When we worship God, He does amazing things. When I became a Christ-follower, I was part of a small church that had three meetings a week. Don't faint! Yes, three church meetings a week. They could have had ten and I still would have been at them all, singing and praising God. I wanted to praise Him, but more than that, I needed to praise Him. And let me give you a little perspective on this: I can't sing! In fact, my voice makes the little penguin in Happy Feet sound like Elvis. When God handed out smooth voices, He gave me a cheese grater. My amazing musician brother-in-law described my voice as the sound of constant modulation. I took it as a compliment.

We lived for about six years in the beautiful city of Ballarat, Victoria. In front of our usual seat at church sat two young girls named Fiona and Maree. They could both sing and play musical instruments. At times I would hit notes that had yet to be discovered. Car alarms would go off, ships would crash against rocks and mothers would take their children off the street. These notes would cause these two young girls to turn and look back, thinking there was someone strangling a cat. I'd smile and say, "You complain, I'll sing louder." They wouldn't say anything! They were very gracious. I may not be gifted to sing, but I can worship. I have learnt that if I choose to worship and place my focus on God's greatness whether I feel like it or not, it wins battles. The role of worship in overcoming mental anguish cannot be underestimated.

Think about this for a moment. The first thing our enemy will try to do is get us to stop worshipping God. "Stay at home today, you don't feel well enough, no one understands what you're going through... don't go." "Did God really say you needed to go the church and worship with others?" Doubt!

It is amazing what lifting our voices to a loving heavenly Father does to the spirit. When there is nothing worth singing praises about except God then that is enough reason to sing. When my mind would run crazy and thoughts would seek to dominate my mind, I knew I could sing to my God of love and grace. Rather than focus on me and all my faults I could change my focus onto His greatness. It's not natural, it's a choice! Peace would flood my heart and mind.

Isaiah 26:3

You will keep in perfect peace him whose mind is steadfast, because he trusts in you.

The Message version says this:

'People with their minds set on you, you keep completely whole. Steady on their feet, because they keep at it and don't quit. Depend on God and keep at it because in the Lord God you have a sure thing.'

King David, while being pursued by his enemy, sang these words:

Psalm 59:16, 17

But I will sing of your strength, in the morning I will sing of your love; for you are my fortress, my refuge in times of trouble.

O my Strength, I sing praise to you; you, O God, are my fortress, my loving God.

When it comes to worship, will we close our mouths and think that we know better, or will we sing and trust what God says? When we begin to praise Him, He will set ambushes and bring great victories in our lives. These choices made in the everyday grittiness of life make all the difference. These are the 'day in, day out', battles we fight within ourselves. These are the decisions that make us or break us. These are the choices where victories are won or lost. We will face storms in our lives, yet with our steps ordered by the Word of God, we can walk through any storm.

Psalm 37:23 (NLT)

The lord directs the steps of the godly. He delights in every detail of their lives.

When we choose to simply believe God in His goodness and mercy, trusting His word as the ultimate authority in our lives and actions, we will start to win battles and overcome enemies. When we worship though we don't feel like it, when we trust God's thinking over our thoughts, and fight our fights by His battle plans, we will see real change in our circumstances. In doing this, we will climb higher, reach further, and achieve more. The fog lifts, the sky clears and we can see clearly again. Breathe the air of this new place. The place is called 'life beyond depression and mental illness' and the view from there truly is spectacular.

NOT AN OPTIONAL EXTRA

STEP 7: BREAKING FREE OF REGRET

First things first: if anyone says that forgiveness is easy, they probably never had anything to forgive. Forgiveness can be one of the hardest things to do; however, it certainly is one of the most vital! Secondly, some people will never ask for our forgiveness, and they will certainly never deserve forgiveness.

As we go through this section, I believe that there are people who are reading these words, who will find freedom from past events that have kept them tied up in knots for years. There is no way to overestimate the importance of what we are about to cover.

I believe passionately in what I call 'clean slate living'. This metaphor comes from the days when you could go to a bar, or even a corner store without cash on you, and the shop keeper would keep a tab or slate. Every time you had a drink or bought something, the bartender or shop owner put the amount of the purchase on your slate. Farmers had a slate at the local stores and when the crop was harvested, they 'cleaned the slate' by paying for all the goods they had used up until that time.

In life, things build up on our slate, and I firmly believe in living with a clean slate. I think the Bible agrees with me on this when it says,

Forgive us our debts as we forgive those our debtors
Matthew 6:12 (NKJV)

This is cleaning the slate. It is taking anything that has been added to the slate, for example hurts or offences, and wiping it clean ready to start again.

Life is a journey, and as we travel we pick up baggage. Imagine with me for a moment that we go on a flight and get off at the other end but leave the baggage on the plane. The plane takes another trip and another trip, yet none of the baggage ever gets taken off. In a very short time that plane will be too heavy to take off. This can so easily happen in our lives and, in a surprisingly short space of time, we find ourselves stuck on the tarmac taxiing around, unable to fly. The baggage is too heavy and needs to be unloaded. The baggage of past mistakes, the baggage of regrets, the baggage of hurts, the baggage of tragedy and suffering—they are real burdens, but God wants them unloaded so you can fly again.

'Cast *all your anxiety on him, for He cares for you.'*
1 Peter 5:7

If we don't unload we will either crash or never take off. Either way, we are going down, living in a void, perpetually spinning our wheels and going nowhere. Our baggage weighs us down and becomes the object of our thoughts, occupying large amounts of time and energy as we try to process and deal with stuff. Why do you think so many depression and mental health sufferers suffer with exhaustion? It's because it takes a huge amount of energy to continue the destructive thought patterns. If we throw in the emotions of anger, hate, self loathing, misery, guilt, pain, bitterness, sadness, anxiety and any other emotion we can think of, we see a person absolutely exhausted from the turmoil of the mind. I am convinced that mental exhaustion is far more draining than physical exhaustion.

Here's some practical advice; if we are going to get this plane off the ground again, we need to throw the baggage off the plane! We need to wipe the slate clean.

It doesn't matter what metaphor we want to use. What matters is that we reach a point where our hearts and consciences are clear.

FORGIVENESS

One sure journey to a messed up mind and heart, is the road called unforgiveness. Forgiveness is a major part of our healing. I would even go as far as to say that if we refuse to forgive, we will never move to a place beyond the grasp of depression and mental illness. All illnesses of the mind revolve around thoughts. If thoughts are constantly occupied with bitterness and hurt as a result of unforgiveness, the mind cannot move forward toward healing and renewal. I truly believe that there are thousands suffering with depression because of unforgiveness. In fact, unforgiveness could be the single greatest contributing factor to depression and mental illness around our globe.

"I cannot forgive him," "I will not forgive them," and, "I will never forgive myself." How many times do we hear these statements? Don't get me wrong here. I'm not saying that forgiveness is easy. If it were easy then we would not have a problem.

A young woman spent extended periods of time in various mental health care facilities. After being in and out of hospital, she is now heavily medicated and struggling in her life. This young lady truly loves Jesus, and after hearing her story I am surprised that she would love anyone again. If I had hair, it would have gone curly just listening to what she has been through. She struggles to forgive and I don't blame her one bit. In fact, I think that if I had gone through what she has gone through I am confident that, as spiritual as I like to think I am, I would struggle to forgive.

So I'm not saying it's easy, however, it is necessary for recovery. The truth of the matter is that it may take her years to fully forgive those people. It's a journey and what thrills me most is that she has decided to start the journey—not a journey of denial, but a journey of forgiveness and healing.

2 Corinthians 10:3-5

For though we live in the world, we do not wage war as the world does. The weapons we fight with are not the weapons of the world. On the contrary, they have divine power to demolish strongholds. We demolish arguments and every pretension that sets itself up against the knowledge of God, and we take captive every thought to make it obedient to Christ.

TRUSTING AGAIN

It's interesting to note that even non-biblical sources advise that forgiveness is extremely powerful in the healing process. In the light of the verse above, let us look at forgiveness and unforgiveness on a spiritual level.

Let's just take the first part of that verse in relation to forgiveness and unforgiveness: 'For we live in this world.'

This is very true, and stuff happens in this world that is wrong and upsetting. The Message puts it this way;

'T*he world is unprincipled. It's dog-eat-dog out there! The world doesn't fight fair.'*

This world is unprincipled, it is dog-eat-dog, and it certainly doesn't fight fair. So what do we do about that? Do we live in hatred and bitterness with a 'get even' attitude? Do we choose to not forgive? It is a choice! Is this how to live? Is this what God says is the way to a free and fulfilled, abundant life?

'T*he weapons we fight with are not the weapons of the world. On the contrary, they have divine power to* *demolish strongholds.'*

Will we claim to believe *in* God yet not believe He is bigger than the issue at hand or will we choose to simply believe God?

CHOOSING THE FIGHT

We need to understand that we are in a fight. There is a battle for man's soul, and one of the chief weapons used by the enemy is our unforgiveness. Unforgiveness will destroy your soul. It will consume the holder rather than the perpetrator until the unforgiven offence so binds the person that life is not possible without that bitter taste in the mouth.

Unforgiveness will destroy your soul. Yet, if we choose to forgive, no matter how hard and how many times we have to, then we disarm the enemy. That's what it means to use weapons that are mighty and full of divine power to demolish strongholds.

Unforgiveness is a stronghold that needs to be taken down. We must call on divine strength to accomplish this. The power to forgive comes from the power of the great forgiver.

Jesus said, "Father, forgive them."

Actually, it's commanded to forgive. We tend to view a command in a negative way. However, this is a powerfully positive command.

'Forgive others as you have been forgiven'. **Ephesians 4:32**

Let's look at a passage on forgiveness in the light of the question asked earlier; will we be a believer *in* God, or will we believe God? Will we give God's Word the place of ultimate authority in our lives, or only accept His divine words when they fit into how we feel?

The story of the unforgiving servant was sparked by a question asked by one of Jesus' disciples, "How many times do we need to forgive someone?" This is a reasonable question. However Jesus' response to this question leads us to see that Jesus wanted this disciple to see a far greater picture.

Matthew 18:21-35 (MSG)

At that point Peter got up the nerve to ask, 'Master, how many times do I forgive a brother or sister who hurts me? Seven?'

Jesus replied, 'Seven! Hardly. Try seventy times seven.'

The kingdom of God is like a king who decided to square accounts with his servants. As he got under way, one servant was brought before him who had run up a debt of a hundred thousand dollars. He couldn't pay up, so the king ordered the man, along with his wife, children, and goods, to be auctioned off at the slave market.

The poor wretch threw himself at the king's feet and begged, 'Give me a chance and I'll pay it all back.' Touched by his plea, the king let him off, erasing the debt.

The servant was no sooner out of the room when he came upon one of his fellow servants who owed him ten dollars. He seized him by the throat and demanded, 'Pay up. Now!'

The poor wretch threw himself down and begged, 'Give me a chance and I'll pay it all back.' But he wouldn't do it. He had him arrested and put in jail until the debt was paid. When the other servants saw this going on, they were outraged and brought a detailed report to the king.

The king summoned the man and said, 'You evil servant! I forgave your entire debt when you begged me for mercy. Shouldn't you be compelled to be merciful to your fellow servant who asked for mercy?' The king was furious and put the screws to the man until he paid back his entire debt. And that's exactly what my Father in heaven is going to do to each one of you who doesn't forgive unconditionally anyone who asks for mercy.

When I first read this passage I thought, 'What an idiot! How stupid is this man? That's ridiculous to do something like that!' How ridiculous is it that someone would choose to destroy their life over not forgiving a debt that is minuscule, compared to the debt they have been forgiven of?

Uncomfortable? Keep reading, it's important. I've had to really live this one.

Forgiveness starts the process of healing. It gives us freedom to leave our past and step into our future.

We can never move forward if our minds are controlled by the past. It's like we are strapped in a vehicle heading in the wrong direction. We need to stop and unbuckle ourselves, release, get out and start heading in the right direction.

The Bible talks extensively about living with a clean conscience. What's important here is our conscience and thought process—the cleanliness of our minds and hearts. We might say about other people, "How can they live with themselves?" I don't know about someone else. What is important is how we live with ourselves.

This will get tough, but it's important that you continue. On this journey to recovery, it doesn't get more important than this! I read this warning the other day:

2 Timothy 3:1-5

But mark this: There will be terrible times in the last days. People will be lovers of themselves, lovers of money, boastful, proud, abusive, disobedient to their parents, ungrateful, unholy, without love, unforgiving, slanderous, without self-control, brutal, not lovers of the good, treacherous, rash, conceited, lovers of pleasure rather than lovers of God—having a form of godliness but denying its power. Have nothing to do with them.

Note that alongside such things as boastful, proud, disobedient, slanderous, without self-control, brutal, ungrateful and unholy is the word 'unforgiving'.

I wonder, although it probably cannot be proven, if maybe the sudden increase in depression and mental illness in our Western society has a direct correlation to an 'unforgiving' attitude running through our modern culture. Our culture tends to teach that it's all about us and we become self-focused and consumed.

It's interesting to note that the word in this passage for 'unforgiveness', is *aspondos*, referring to 'a state of hostilities and refusal to enter into a covenant'. The King James Version used the word 'trucebreaker'.

2 Timothy 3:1-5 (MSG)

Don't be naive. There are difficult times ahead. As the end approaches, people are going to be self-absorbed, money-hungry, self-promoting, stuck-up, profane, contemptuous of parents, crude, coarse, dog-eat-dog, unbending, slanderers, impulsively wild, savage, cynical, treacherous, ruthless, bloated windbags, addicted to lust, and allergic to God. They'll make a show of religion, but behind the scenes they're animals. Stay clear of these people.

However we look at it, this is a state of defiance toward others and toward God's plan. God instructs us to love our enemies and bless those who curse us. Remember we are talking about living life with a clean slate and taking steps toward a life beyond depression and mental illness. It's a huge step forward to choose what God says over what we think in relation to forgiveness. So today, make a choice with me and, having God as a witness, choose to forgive. It may seem impossible, and you may not even want to, but the right choice *is* very often the one we don't feel like making. With this act of the will, this choice to forgive, comes something liberating. The moist damp limiting grayness associated with the constant churning over and over within our minds begins to clear. Light shines in and, perhaps for the first time in years, we can see beyond the limitations of pain and regrets into a brighter new land of forgiveness.

Luke 6:27, 28

But I tell you who hear me: Love your enemies, do good to those who hate you, bless those who curse you, pray for those who mistreat you.

FORGIVENESS IS NOT AN OPTIONAL EXTRA

Forgiveness starts the process of healing. It gives us freedom to leave our past and step into our future.

Forgiving is not like when we buy a new car and we say, "I'll have the leather trim, those nice alloy wheels, the tinted windows." These are optional extras (well, perhaps not the really cool wheels). The vehicle will run fine with the standard pack. A person won't run at all if there is unforgiveness in their heart. In fact, no one will, believer or non-believer. Unforgiveness is like removing all the electronics from the car. It simply will have no spark or power and will not go anywhere. It may sit there and look the part from the outside, and no one will notice while the outside is polished up and looking fine. But the vehicle isn't going anywhere while unforgiveness is there! Unforgiveness will stop a person moving forward into maturity. To be stuck in the garage, never moving forward because of bitterness is sad and contrary to God's word and great plan for our lives. With unforgiveness within us, how can we fulfill the caring for others, feeding the hungry, clothing the naked and visiting the sick that is talked about in Matthew chapter 25?

To be non-forgiving is to destroy the very foundation of Christ in our lives. I certainly am not here to judge anyone. There are so many who have gone through such horrific things that I'm not pointing the finger at anyone. If I'm pointing at all, I hope I'm pointing toward God's word so that each of us will see that however hard and painful forgiving can be, it is vital to us all if we are to move forward.

Why? Because freedom to live comes when we forgive!

I find it hard to believe that anybody could live beyond depression and mental illness while still caught in the bitter cycle of unforgiveness.

Here is a story of forgiveness from my life. These incidents happened over a period of almost a decade. What was more important then what happened with that person, was what was happening in me. I bring this example up because over this period I was subjected to what could only, in my view, be described as spiritual abuse. It wasn't physical in any way, but rather emotional bullying and intimidation by a person senior to me whom I respected greatly and still do respect and love.

For some people, constant belittlement and criticism has little effect, but for someone like me who was coming out of depression and mental illness, the environment was very difficult. Bombarded with comments that always implied 'you're never good enough', everything I did was criticized, and very often in a harsh, aggressive yelling manner. The worst thing was the inconsistency. In a moment, conversation with this person could change from constructive, level and reasonable to outright abusive without reason. Needless to say, these were very difficult years. I did learn many good things that have helped me as well. There certainly was some gold in a huge mountain of rubble. In fact, it is probably the greatest example in my personal life of Romans 8:28.

Romans 8:28 (NASB)

And we know that God causes all things to work together for good to those who love God, to those who are called according to His purpose.

I learned that although God may not cause certain things to happen, He certainly does cause them to turn into things that work for good in our lives, including bad things. There is a proviso with this verse, and that is, that we live with a pure heart to God. I don't believe that anything can work for good if we remain caught in the downward spiral of bitterness and unforgiveness. If we refuse to forgive I think it is ludicrous for us to expect this working for good in our lives.

For a long time I could not forgive this person and you might think, "Well, some spiritual guru you are!" I guess the good thing is that I've never considered myself a guru... just as well!

The results of living that way were real. This is what would happen. I would forgive him and it would be alright for a while until the thoughts would come back and the bitterness would rise up. I would have to stop myself and forgive him all over again. The results of unforgiveness in my life were a loss of joy and wonder in Christ. Oh yeah, I still looked the part. I could still preach and do the regular stuff required, and I was still genuine about serving Christ with all I had. However, that inward mindset brought about a loss of genuine happiness and a falling back into depressive behavior. It all became very shallow and hard. My heart became calloused and eventually I shut down toward this person. I put everything he said aside, and dismissed it as the rambling of a bully. I didn't want to be hurt anymore.

The strange thing is, I became very religious and judgmental of others. My heart that lived for others and loving them became more and more inwardly focused and concerned for the trap I saw myself in. My thought life went from outward to inward, from an outward person trying to help others, to an inward-thinking, self-consumed person. I didn't mean to—it just happened and this unforgiveness was a large part of it. I was going to say that I was serving God with all my heart. However, when I think about it, if I don't forgive someone, then part of my heart is occupied constantly with the bitterness of an unresolved hurt rather than serving God.

I cannot say the exact point where I finally forgave him. I had to forgive him many, many times during these difficult years. There was a change in my heart after many times of forgiving him. I don't know when I did it; however I do know I have forgiven him. I can tell this because whenever I think of situations that happened or I'm in conversations where the events from that time are mentioned, there is no bitterness and anger anymore. In fact, and here is a weird thing, the bitterness has been replaced with a genuine love and care for that person, and sympathy for what led him to be that kind of man.

Someone once described not forgiving as burning down your own house to spite someone else. Today let forgiveness reign in our lives and start anew.

Martin Luther King said, "We must develop and maintain the capacity to forgive. He who is devoid of the power to forgive is devoid of the power to love."

And again, "Forgiveness is not an occasional act; it is a permanent attitude."

Forgiveness is a gift. It's a choice that goes against the hurt in our lives.

PULLING THE WEEDS OUT

As a gardener, I'm pathetic! Honestly terrible. I do however have a particular skill in growing weeds. In fact, I'm very proficient at mowing over weeds. This works well, and everything looks fine for a few days. The problem is that the root of the weed is still there and it grows again. Also in my mowing, I chop off the top of the weed and manage to spread it over other parts of the lawn and in turn, I get weeds growing there as well. Don't we do this in life? We chop the tops off so that when visitors come round they don't see the bitterness. We can even forget about it for a short while. However, weeds grow again as bitterness rears its ugly head.

The only way to successfully get rid of weeds is to pull them out and to get rid of the root. The Bible talks about 'a root of bitterness.' The only way to remove the root is to dig it out with forgiveness!

Hebrews 12:15 (NLT)

Look after each other so that none of you fails to receive the grace of God. Watch out that no poisonous root of bitterness grows up to trouble you, corrupting many.

In all aspects of our lives, we need to simply believe God and take Him at His Word. His Word is true and sets a person free. Let us be very real and open with ourselves. Let us ask the question, "have I been putting what I think above or before what God says in His word?" If this is true, then it's time to clean the slate and start again. It's time to obey His word over our thoughts.

Everybody needs to face times in their lives where forgiveness is chosen over unforgiveness. Is it your time today?

Who do you need to forgive? Or who do you need to ask forgiveness of? Let us face the truth, that unforgiveness will block the road to recovery. It's time! Today is your day to choose to forgive!

I implore, beg, and plead you to stop reading now and clean the state. Yes, I know you will have to fight those thoughts again, but I believe you can, by God's grace and power, demolish this stronghold. Read this verse again as we close this chapter and open up our lives to a new life. Freedom is what every human heart desires.

Forgiveness will grant you that freedom.

2 Corinthians 10:3-5

For though we live in the world, we do not wage war as the world does. The weapons we fight with are not the weapons of the world. On the contrary, they have divine power to demolish strongholds. We demolish arguments and every pretension that sets itself up against the knowledge of God, and we take captive every thought to make it obedient to Christ.

YOU CAN RESCUE FANTASIA

STEP 8: UNDERSTANDING OUR GREATEST ABILITY

I'm a runner. I've always been a runner. I don't know when I started running, but from a very young age I've been a runner. Now let me clarify this statement so I don't give a false impression. If all this running was done physically, I would be able to run marathons without breaking a sweat. I'm a runner because ever since I can remember, I've run from my problems.

We have a drug and alcohol rehabilitation facility about 30 kilometers from where we live. It's called Sherwood Cliffs and it has the most astounding results with a success rate second to none for people who stay for the whole program. I believe that over 90 percent of the people who go through the program never return to drug and alcohol dependency. Some, however, choose not to stay for the whole program because it becomes too confronting and they run. They run from the facility and from the people trying to help them, and virtually always run back into drug and alcohol abuse.

This chapter will get confronting. At times you may want to throw the book across the room and you'll wonder how I know you so well. It's not that I know you, it's just that I've come to know what we all do when we struggle with depression and mental illness. I want, with all my heart, to help each and every person who read these pages to get beyond the debilitating effects of depression and of mental illness. It will take courage to keep going, but keep going we must. Victory awaits and you have already come so far. I'm so proud that you are taking these steps, so keep stepping forward with me. To get this far proves to me that you have the faith for this!

THE NEVERENDING STORY

The classic tale *The Neverending Story* is a tale of courage, set in Fantasia, a mythical land where peace reigned until 'the Nothing' started to destroy everything in its path. Nothing could stand against the Nothing. But there was hope, found in a young warrior named Atreyu, who had to overcome many obstacles in the race to save Fantasia. In one task he walked between two great monoliths that could have killed him in an instant; the remains of many others lay all around him. This he accomplished, yet, before him was the most difficult task of all. If he failed, the world would be lost, and all would fall into the darkness that was consuming everything.

Atreyu walked and walked and there in the midst of a blizzard, came across a mirror. In this mirror he had to stare at the thing that many of us find the most frightening sight of all. He had to look at himself, and not just at himself but within himself, staring at the real core of who he was.

What is our task in this chapter? You guessed it. You and I have to be able to stare at our reflection, see ourselves for who we really are, and choose not to run from what we see. To simply own who we are can be a frightening thing. I told you this chapter will get confronting. I want you to trust me now. I will be alongside you every step through these pages. Remember, I've lived this stuff, and I care enough to say what needs saying. Why? Because what we are about to get into is truly life-changing. It's where the tide turns. It's the place where a choice makes a massive difference.

Think of it this way: we're on one side of a huge bridge. Below is a great chasm of all our doubts and fears. All the "I can never change, I'm no good, I've messed up too many times" rubbish from our minds is there below calling out. The mistakes of the past are all there, and every time we get close to crossing the bridge we see the depth of the chasm, and all the regrets and fears of the years past. They are there and they are real, let's not deny that.

It may not help to imagine the bridge as being a swing bridge straight out of an Indiana Jones movie. Most of us would think, 'I'm not going across that'. Let me assure you that this bridge is completely safe. It will not look or feel safe, but it is perfectly safe. It is strengthened by the very power of God. It has divine power set in place to make it possible for you and me to cross.

On the other side of the bridge is a world very different from the confines of depression, bipolar disorder and the like. It is a world where our thoughts don't keep us up all night, where rest is beautiful and where peace reigns. It is a place where life's challenges still exist of course; not everything is perfect. However, life is not bound by a neverending series of painful situations, or the all-consuming nothingness of an existence void of life. It's a place of security and wonder, hope and peace. I live there now and I want you to imagine me standing at the other side of the bridge calling you across, encouraging you to see that the journey is worth every nervous step. Actually, I don't mind if you imagine me standing next to you holding your hand and walking across with you. Just know this: with every fiber of my being, I know you need to take responsibility and cross this bridge and if I can help you across, I will.

I've walked this bridge and yes, it looks scary. It even feels shaky, but that's just us. There is a Chinese proverb that goes like this: "A journey of a thousand miles begins with a single step." With all my heart I want you to take these steps. You're already further across than you think.

The choice is not to run anymore, but rather to step into responsibility.

STEPPING OUT OF THE FAMILIAR

Familiar environments, whether beneficial or destructive, can become a security. But they can also become a cage that stops us from reaching places of freedom. Long term depression or mental illness can become a security to the sufferer. It gives reasons, and sometimes excuses as well. Sometimes these reasons are entirely valid. However, here lies the issue; a person in a cycle of depression or mental illness produces a set of reactionary responses, or 'survival mechanisms' to given sets of stimuli. We all have these sets of coping responses. These are coping mechanisms that are used to handle life's situations. For instance, one of the most common behaviors is isolationism—cutting ourselves off from society.

Here's an example to explain my point: This situation happened a number of years ago with a friend of mine. This person suffered from depression and had done for years. On anti-depressant medication, my friend was quite stable. However, life, with all its twists, ups, and downs, would become difficult at times, as it does for everybody. My friend's response was to consciously (and she knew exactly what would happen) stop taking her medication. She did this knowing that the result would end up being a trip to the hospital and a few weeks of observation in the psych ward. Perhaps the first time she went in, it was the best thing for my friend, and maybe even the second time. However, this learned behavior or patterning became a response that she used to blame others and escape reality and responsibility for a while.

I will never forget the day I made my observation to my friend in the psych ward. Her reaction was that of a person who thought that no one knew and she had just been found out. What was so sad about the whole situation was that this wonderful person and personal friend chose to keep running and not take this step toward recovery. I know some will say, "She couldn't help it," and, "Hospital is the best place for that person." Sometimes that is right for a season. However, if the only result is a repeat episode six months later, we have a wrong understanding of this illness and the road to recovery.

In this case, and I am purposefully not generalizing, the doctors had done everything they could. She herself chose this course of action and ran away. It seemed easier to generate a manic episode by refusing to take the medication, than to take responsibility and keep living though the challenging situations.

I understand completely the desire to run, but there are better ways to cope. Yes, they are ways that will involve challenge, but they will also lead to healing.

The end result must be healing. The steps in this book all lead toward freedom. Here is a point where a clash between me and the medical professions is possible. I'm a huge believer in the medical profession. I believe that medication for mental and emotional issues is a reasonable response to help people cope for a time. However, I also believe that God works in people in order to produce a better life—a life full and free, a life beyond the grasp of depression and mental illness. I believe a productive and wonderful life is available for everyone. As I stated earlier, even if that picture does include medication, it's okay, as long as the journey is heading toward freedom. The issue I have is with the attitude that says 'because someone suffers from mental illness now, that there is nothing they can do, and they just have to come to terms with this condition for the rest of their life'. This, I believe, is a wrong understanding and one of the most devastating effects of this thinking is the total destruction of hope. Even if a bipolar sufferer has to take medication for the rest of their lives, I firmly believe that they can become an active and productive member of society. Their life is of tremendous value and there is a reason for their existence. There is great hope for a better life. When hope is lost, the reason for living dies and thus we end up with high levels of hopelessness, depression and suicide within western culture.

THE FAMILIAR BECOMES A CRUTCH

Let's look at another person I have known. This long term depression and mental illness sufferer responded well to friendship and care, counseling sessions and visits, and had a group of wonderful caring people helping him. This person became better and better over a long period, until he reached the point where he could slowly begin to enter back into society. (Bear in mind this person had received a disability pension for his mental illness for years.)

At the point where he could have crossed that bridge to a far better place, with a team of caring people around him to help him every step of the way, he chose not to take responsibility for his actions. To make the right choice would have meant finding work and gradually, but eventually, letting his government payments reduce. He chose to blame his condition because he didn't want to forgo his government handout payments. He chose a half-existence, rather than a better life. He ran from the opportunity to leave the cycle of self destruction and made a bad choice. The crazy thing is that he was already halfway across the bridge to recovery when he turned back. This could have been the final step across this bridge for him but he didn't want to take responsibility for the choice he knew he needed to make.

This person made a conscious choice, valuing his government payment more than his recovery. He ran at the moment of hope and ended up going so far to prove he needed the payment that he ran back to alcohol and substance abuse. He is now still living in a cycle of excuse, running from responsibility.

God would have helped him and people would have helped

him, however there are times when we need to actually help ourselves by making right choices.

I understand this fear of getting back into society. I have sat in cars outside houses, unable to move my legs for fear, so gripped by all my past thoughts and fears that I was paralyzed. As hard as it is, it must be done. We have to take responsibility for who we are right now—not our good intentions, nor our crushed dreams, our hopes, or our anything, just who we are right now.

When we look at the children of Israel after they decided not to enter the promised land, we can learn some valuable lessons. History shows that this nation came out of slavery in Egypt with God leading them through a desolate place to reach the promised land. Yet when they arrived at the point of going into the land, they didn't. What happened was that they sent twelve spies in who checked out the land. When they returned, two gave a good report. "It will be tough, but we can, by God's strength, take this land." The other ten were negative and focused on how difficult it would be. The people went with the negative report. The result was a 40-year stint of wandering around the wilderness, going nowhere fast. Millions died, and the result was that 40 years later they came back to the same place and had the same choice to make. Will we trust God and go into the promised land, or will we continue in a half-existence in the desolate places?

Here are some observations. You can find the story in the book of Numbers 13 and 14. The story is far too long to put in here however I encourage you to read it.

The wilderness or desolate places were never to be their final destination. Yet millions died there, never crossing into the promises of God. Let's make this personal. Depression and mental illness are not designed to be the desolate place we exist in forever. It may be a place we are traveling in and through but God has a promised land for you. And just like these people had to cross the Jordan River to get into the promised land, we must take responsibility for our actions and choose to cross as well.

God sustained them through the time in the wilderness and 'through' is the important word here. They were designed to go through, not live in, the desert places. We are designed to enter a promised land. Of course, this promised land is not some sort of spiritual Christian 'nirvana' where there is never a problem. While we have breath in our lungs, we will have difficulties. It's part of the human condition. In fact, the Bible tells us that *'man is born for trouble, as surely as sparks fly upward.'* **Job 5:7** We do go through trouble and desolate places. But we were designed to go through them and grow through them, not set up permanent residence in them.

One of the world's favorite Psalms was written by King David, who said, "Though I walk through the valley of the shadow of death," not, "This valley will always be my home."

Recovery is in the choices we make. It is our choice and our choice alone to get well. It will not be instant. It's a walking from one land to another but we must reach the point where although we can blame someone else for our troubles, we choose not to any more. Yes, things have happened, and many very hurtful things take place in our society. These things involve other people's influence and fault, however the choice as to where we go from here is all ours to make. It's not easy but it's very necessary.

The stories about the escape from Egypt always used to amaze me. The Israelites saw far greater things than I have seen—the Red Sea parting, the plagues in Egypt and the miraculous workings of the hand of God. Yet every time there was an issue, they thought 'We would have been better off in Egypt'. Why did they want to go back when God was moving them forward into a far better place—a place of promise rather than a prison. It's the same in our prison system today. People will reoffend in order to be sent back to prison. Why do they do this? Because the familiar, even when it's a cage, sometimes seems easier than the unknown of the new life outside the prison gate. People think, 'I have my three meals a day, I know this system, and at least I can function in it'. Isn't this the same thing as my friend with the government pension? We who live in a western society should be so thankful for the provision of health services and finances that allow a recovery time. But these things are not meant for us to exist within, but rather to be a help during the passage from desert to a better land. While we can exist for a time in prison, it's not living, and it certainly isn't a great life of wonder and joy.

You and I were designed for the promised land. Our basic need as human beings is to be free! Enslaved people throughout the centuries have fought for freedom. Freedom must be a goal and desire!

The Israelites spent 40 years in their self-imposed wilderness, and God cared for them until He bought them back to the same place, with the same choice to make about leaving the desert and entering into the promises of God. How many of us waste years wandering in dry places spiritually, emotionally and mentally when across the way a far better land is prepared for us? You might see now that you have come to this place before and turned back, only to find that the desert places have become your home. This time, choose the better way—God's way. The way of honesty and responsibility.

OWNING NOW

Let us look at owning today. We cannot do anything about yesterday and we can't change tomorrow, as we cannot know what the future will hold. What we have is today and we do have the ability to own it.

Let's look at another biblical example of a situation that illustrates this very important point. Jacob had spent years running. He had run from his brother after stealing his birthright. Jacob means 'heel-grabber' and he spent years living up to his name. Jacob was a liar, a cheat and a swindler.

Now Jacob was not anti-God or lacking understanding of God.

He had seen visions of angels ascending and descending from heaven. But he came to a point where he could not fix everything by his cunning. By himself, he couldn't work the mess he was in to bring about the right outcome. He came to a point where he decided not to run anymore. Even though Jacob was a very successful man and could be regarded as a high achiever in life, he still had to come to this point—the point of asking, "Will I own who I am and take responsibility for my own actions, or will I keep running?"

Jacob finds himself heading back to his homeland, to a brother from whom he had stolen and whom he had cheated out of something great. We pick up the story here and find Jacob on the journey with all his wives, children, associates and herds.

Genesis 32:23-32 (NASB)

He took them and sent them across the stream. And he sent across whatever he had.

Then Jacob was left alone, and a man wrestled with him until daybreak.

When he saw that he had not prevailed against him, he touched the socket of his thigh; so the socket of Jacob's thigh was dislocated while he wrestled with him.

Then he said, "Let me go, for the dawn is breaking." But he said, "I will not let you go unless you bless me."

So he said to him, "What is your name?" And he said, "Jacob."

He said, "Your name shall no longer be Jacob, but Israel; for you have striven with God and with men and have prevailed."

Then Jacob asked him and said, "Please tell me your name." But he said, "Why is it that you ask my name?" And he blessed him there.

So Jacob named the place Peniel, for he said, "I have seen God face to face, yet my life has been preserved."

Now the sun rose upon him just as he crossed over Peniel, and he was limping on his thigh.

Therefore, to this day the sons of Israel do not eat the sinew of the hip which is on the socket of the thigh, because he touched the socket of Jacob's thigh in the sinew of the hip.

Jacob positioned himself away from everything and got alone with God. The Bible says he wrestled with God for hour after hour after hour. Does that sound familiar? Oh yeah! We can see he wanted to walk a different road. We can see his determination by his persistence. (By getting as far as you have through this book, shows me that you're perhaps just like Jacob, really wanting change, and I congratulate you for this. Let's keep going.) So this wrestling bout continued, World Series Wrestling style, slamming against the ropes, smashing chairs over his opponents head. Well perhaps not quite like that!

Then the one Jacob is wrestling with says, "Let me go, it's time for a new day." Jacob replies, "No way man, I will not let you go until a change happens in my life." (This is the RGV Bible—Revised Gary Version.)

Then the most amazing thing happens. The God figure in this passage asks one of the most simple, yet profound questions ever asked: "What is your name?" Now, think about this. He would have already known Jacob's name, so why ask? Well in those days and in that culture, a name meant so much more than it does in our western culture. The name was not just what a person was called, but rather who they were. Jacob had to come to the point of owning who he was.

What did Jacob actually say when he replied? "I am Jacob." At this point, he chose to own who he was probably for the first time in his life—to own all of it. "Here I am Lord, Jacob. My past, my mistakes, all of it, 'warts and all'. That's me, Jacob the Heel-Grabber."

What's your name? Is it Lonely, Hurt or Messed Up? Is your name Broken or Overwhelmed? Maybe it's Runner or Self-Loathing or even Shame or Angry and I Don't Even Know Why or Hate, Unforgiveness or Bitterness, Depression, Doubt or Fear. It could be all of the above, but whatever it is, when Jacob owned it all, something brilliant happened. God changed his name. Jacob had stopped running. There was no more pretending or faking—I am who I am. That was the point where his name was changed, where Jacob became Israel and where a nation was birthed.

Everything changed that day for Jacob. He still had battles, he still didn't get it right all the time and he was still anything but perfect, but he was changed, and he had taken a huge step forward in becoming everything he was born to be. He had taken responsibility and was stepping across the bridge.

After this moment of ownership, the sun rose on a new day. Even more than that, the sun rose on a new life and on a new man who had truly faced something he had never faced before and who had owned who he was. In one glorious moment, this runner stopped running. He looked in the mirror and owned who he was. He didn't like it but at least it was his. He took responsibility for it all, and that is where it changed.

We all must reach a point where we own who we are.

For most of us, that is not a nice experience. Nice or not, it is necessary for recovery. Even to own where we are is important. Yes, bad things have happened and things will not always be sunshine and roses. Yes, life has been cruel. Yes, things are not the way I planned, and yes, I don't look like Brad Pitt. Hey, it's true! But I am who I am, and until I own at least that, I cannot move forward.

LIMPING BRILLIANTLY

Before we leave Jacob, now named Israel, let's just look at a fascinating thing that happened during the wrestling with God. God did something that would seem totally out of character.

Genesis 32: 24, 31-32

...he touched his hip socket, and Jacob's hip was put out of joint as he wrestled with him... The sun rose upon him as he passed Peniel, limping because of his hip. Therefore to this day the people of Israel do not eat the sinew of the thigh that is on the hip socket, because he touched the socket of Jacob's hip on the sinew of the thigh.

How would you like to pull a great wrestling move that a whole nation recognizes? Isn't it interesting that even though Jacob got a new name and a new life, he was left with a limp for the rest of his days? A physical limp—an injury caused by God's touch and a reminder for him that he wrestled with God and prevailed. Why would God do this? Why would God cripple someone? I think God would much rather we have great character and walk with a limp, than be perfect in a natural way and have a flawed character.

I don't think Jacob would have traded his limp for anything. It would have caused him pain and possibly led to a bad back and headaches but I don't think he would have traded it even if he had the opportunity. This limp would have become precious to him as every step and every hobble would be a reminder of the touch of God. Imagine Jacob meeting someone in church today. They might say, "What's wrong with you?" or, "Come and I'll pray for you. 'Lay hands on the sick and they will recover'. "No," would probably be Jacob's reply. "I've already had hands laid on me. This limp came from the hand of God himself. This limp is my mark; it's my sign and my constant reminder of God's interaction and intimacy in my life. Yes, I walk differently now! Not just my walk, but my life is different. My name is different and my future is new. This limp is my evidence of this change. With every step, I'm reminded of God's touch, and I will not let you take that from me. I remember every step that night, the wrestling, the old, the new, the fact that God met me at my point of greatest need and touched and changed me. When all else is aside and here I am limping along in my human state, I can remember that the almighty hands of a loving God surround me. In my limp, I know I have seen the face of God."

MY BRILLIANT LIMP

My mind has caused me great pain for years and yet today I wouldn't change it for anything. It's my mark, my constant reminder of the touch of God. You cannot take that from me. I know God so much better for the pain of my journey, my limp.

Job said toward the end of his suffering, *"My ears had heard of you, but now my eyes have seen you."* **Job 42:5** I have seen Him in the battle, in the dark where He has shown that even darkness is as light to Him. He has stood beside me and has been my help in time of need. I have come through the desert leaning on my lover.

Song of Solomon 8:3 (KJV)

Who is this that cometh up from the wilderness, leaning upon her beloved?

Here are some passages that have meant a huge amount to me over the years. There are passages in the Bible that mean so much more to certain people, simply because of what they have had to live through. There is a verse in Jude that is that way for me.

Jude 1:24

To him who is able to keep you from falling and to present you before his glorious presence without fault and with great joy.

He keeps me from falling. As we step into responsibility, He steps up *His* responsibility to keep us from falling. Here are some others to encourage us.

2 Timothy 1:12b

'Because I know whom I have believed, and am convinced that he is able to guard what I have entrusted to him for that day.'

Hebrews 2:18

Because he himself suffered when he was tempted, he is able to help those who are being tempted

Notice the '*He is able*' parts.

Ephesians 6:13

Therefore put on the full armor of God, so that when the day of evil comes, you may be able to stand your ground, and after you have done everything, to stand.

Psalm 37:31 (NASB)

The law of his God is in his heart; His steps do not slip.

Ephesians 3:20

Now to him who is able to do immeasurably more than all we ask or imagine, according to his power that is at work within us.

God is able to do 'immeasurably more', or 'exceedingly abundantly above all.'

Ephesians 3:20 (MSG)

God can do anything, you know—far more than you could ever imagine or guess or request in your wildest dreams!

Ephesians 3:20 (KJV)

Now unto him that is able to do exceeding abundantly above all that we ask or think, according to the power that worketh in us.

This is where the miraculous happens. When we take responsibility and own who we are, God intervenes with his limitless power that is able to work in us for a greater life and future.

'OUT OF SIGHT—DYNAMITE'

What does 'immeasurably more' or 'exceedingly abundantly' actually mean? To find the meaning we need to examine a few Greek words. 'Able' is the Greek word *dunamai*, meaning 'capable, strong and powerful'.

'Immeasurably more' means 'above the above or beyond: relating to a country of residence lying beyond our own borders'.

'Power' is *dunamis,* where we get our word 'dynamite', and 'works' is *energeo* from which we get 'energy'.

So we could read this passage like this:

'To God, who is capable, strong and powerful to do above and even 'above the above' of anything we can imagine or ask, this is according to His active, dynamite energy at work within us.'

So we see that God has this incredibly great power, and He is capable of doing above the above when it comes to us and our fight to be free.

What if we are stopping the power of God moving in our lives?

In the previous chapter we discussed forgiveness, mainly focusing on how we must forgive others. While we are on the subject of taking responsibility, let's cover when *we* need forgiveness. Someone once said, "If I could kick the person most responsible for my troubles, I wouldn't be able to sit down for a month." We all sin, and we all have sinned. The Bible tells us that *'we have all sinned and fallen short of the glory of God.'*

Romans 3:23

The Bible also says that *'if we confess our sins he is faithful and just to forgive our sins and purify us from all unrighteousness.'* **1 John 1:9**

LAYING IT ALL ON THE TABLE TODAY

Let nothing be hidden anymore. No secrets, no hiding. No running off and hiding in the bush like Adam did after he sinned, then trying to blame it on his wife, "It's this woman you gave me, Lord." Remember, this is the beginning of a brand new day and we, like Jacob, have to own what we are and what we have become. I'm convinced that God is able! He is able to forgive us no matter what. He will choose grace all the time toward us if our hearts are open to Him.

There is destiny in this; beside human error, beside faults and failings, beside broken marriages and wayward children, beside bankruptcy and business ventures, God will use every bit of it, if we are willing, to produce something beautiful in its time, even if where we are now is not what we would consider to be the optimum plan God has or has had for our lives.

As we close this chapter, I would like to give you a bit of homework.

There is an incredible illustration of this profound principle found in the Old Testament. King David, who wrote some of the most loved biblical passages of all time and who was known as a man after the heart of God, made a bad choice. He lusted after someone else's wife, slept with her, made her pregnant and then to cover his wickedness did some pretty evil stuff including murdering the woman's husband.

You can read the passages in 2 Samuel chapters 11 and 12. Here is an amazing thing; out of this seemingly disastrous relationship came the next king of Israel, a young man named

Solomon who did amazing things for God and for all time will be known as the wisest man to ever live.

This story graphically illustrates that good can come from the most treacherous and adverse situations. This true story involves wickedness, crime, deceit, lust, drunkenness, murder and loss, but also repentance, new beginnings and, most of all, God's incredible love toward people.

David, like all of us, came to a point of destiny when he had a choice. That choice was to own himself right where he was. He had to throw out the blame game, dispel all excuses and take responsibility for whom and what he had become. Great and defining moments are these ones.

OUR GREATEST ABILITY IS RESPONSIBILITY

Right now is the time, as this chapter closes. Let us all choose to own who we are right now. It's in doing this that we allow a better future into the equation of our lives.

Can you answer this question: "What is your name?"

ISOLATION = DEVASTATION

STEP 9: LEARNING NOT TO WALK ALONE

A bricklayer needed to move 5,000 pounds of bricks from the top of a four storey building to the footpath below.

On an insurance claim form he explained it this way:

"It would have taken too long to carry the bricks down by hand, so I decided to put them in a barrel and lower them by a pulley which I had fastened to the top of the building. After tying the rope securely at ground level, I then went to the top of the building, fastened the rope around the barrel, loaded it with the bricks, and swung it out over the side for the descent.

Then I went down to the sidewalk and untied the rope, holding it securely to guide the barrel down slowly. But since I weigh only 140 pounds, the 500-pound load jerked me off the ground so fast I didn't have time to think of letting go of the rope.

As I passed between the second and third floors, I met the barrel coming down. This accounts for the bruises and lacerations to my upper body. I held tightly to the rope until I reached the top, where my hand became jammed in the pulley. This accounts for my broken thumb. At the same time however, the barrel hit the sidewalk with a bang and the bottom fell out. With the weight of the bricks gone, the barrel weighed only 40 pounds. Thus my 140-pound body began a swift descent and I met the empty barrel coming up. This accounts for my broken ankle.

Slowed only slightly, I continued the descent and landed on the pile of bricks. This accounts for my sprained back and broken collar bone. At this point, I lost my presence of mind completely and let go of the rope. The empty barrel came crashing down on me. This accounts for my head injuries. As to the last question on the form, "What would you do if the same situation arose again?"...Please be advised that I am finished trying to do the job alone."

The Bible tells us this:

Ecclesiastes 4:12

Two are better than one, because they have a good return for their work:

If one falls down, his friend can help him up. But pity the man who falls and has no one to help him up!

Also, if two lie down together, they will keep warm. But how can one keep warm alone?

Though one may be overpowered, two can defend themselves. A cord of three strands is not quickly broken.

Ecclesiastes 4:9-12 (NLT)

A person standing alone can be attacked and defeated, but two can stand back-to-back and conquer. Three are even better, for a triple-braided cord is not easily broken.

WE NEED OTHER PEOPLE

I know they can be annoying, lack understanding and be selfish and irritating at times, but as humans we're designed to do life together, especially when it comes to moving through, and eventually living a life beyond, the confines of depression and mental illness. We need others to help us through. Sorry, but doing it alone just doesn't work!

"But it can be so hard." Yes.

"People just don't understand." Yes, however, we would all be surprised how many actually do.

"I just have to face this myself." It's easy to think that way, but has it helped before? I sincerely doubt it.

"I don't fit in." Does anybody?

The Bible makes these statements, so God is saying directly to each one of us, 'A person standing alone can be attacked and defeated'. Don't try to do it alone. The classic case of a person struggling with their thought life is they choose to isolate themselves from people who can help, yet in the process the fog becomes denser and denser, their thoughts get them even more alone, visibility vanishes and thus the thought life dominates. Hour after hour is spent in thought. It does not help. In fact, it is one of the most self-destructive things we can do.

The war is won when we are either defeated or able to defend ourselves. God states we cannot defend ourselves alone.

I love a good documentary. In Africa, the wild buffalo are about to cross an open plain and the lions are stalking, waiting for the right moment to attack. The lions know that the pack is too strong and they could be trampled if they try to grab a beast from within the pack. So they watch and wait, ever creeping closer and closer. Then they spot a young calf just that little bit behind the rest of the herd. Within moments, the lions cut off the way back to the herd for protection, and come in for the kill. The Bible does give us an idea how these things work, and refers to our evil enemy as a roaring lion.

1 Peter 5:8-11 (MSG)

Keep a cool head. Stay alert. The Devil is poised to pounce, and would like nothing better than to catch you napping. Keep your guard up. You're not the only ones plunged into these hard times. It's the same with Christians all over the world. So keep a firm grip on the faith. The suffering won't last forever. It won't be long before this generous God who has great plans for us in Christ—eternal and glorious plans they are!—will have you put together and on your feet for good. He gets the last word; yes, he does.

1 Peter 5:8 (NLT)

Stay alert! Watch out for your great enemy, the devil. He prowls around like a roaring lion, looking for someone to devour.

Alone we are so vulnerable. Together we can defend ourselves. Whatever you do, don't think you can conquer this thing alone. It is simply not true.

ISOLATION = DEVASTATION

Look at the picture language in this passage:

Ecclesiastes 4:9-12

Verse 9: Together we get a better return for our efforts.

Verse 10: If we fall alone we generally stay down, where a friend can help us up again.

Verse 11: It's cold alone and how true that is! Yet with another we are kept warm.

Verse 12: Alone we can be overcome, but together we are stronger and able to defend ourselves.

GOD DESIGNED US TO FUNCTION TOGETHER.

God made this statement back in the very beginning of creation: *'It is not good for man to be alone'*. **Genesis 2:18**

The need for others and mainly the need for a relationship with Christ are vital to our recovery.

God designed us to be connected to other people and to Him, and the fact that we are not leads us into a minefield of difficulty that results in so much suffering.

When times are tough, the first thing most people do when they are suffering with mental or emotional illnesses is to isolate themselves from the very people they need to be around. What do I mean by the people we need to be around? For instance, a group of people is all a church really is—it's a group of people serving God and growing together. I'll let you in on a secret about churches. There is not one single person who is perfect in any of them, and that is great. The people we need to be around to help us are the ones who are real about their struggles. The benefits of a positive church family environment, a good social club, a strong marriage relationship, or just close, positive friendships, are enormous.

I talk of positive friends, because negative ones can be so destructive. It's called the power of association and we will get to that a little later.

I know I'm laboring this point about isolation and being with other people. It's just that I know how important it is. The Bible backs me up; the very worst thing we can do is isolate ourselves with our thoughts. This will only lead us to deeper depression on a never-ending spiral downwards.

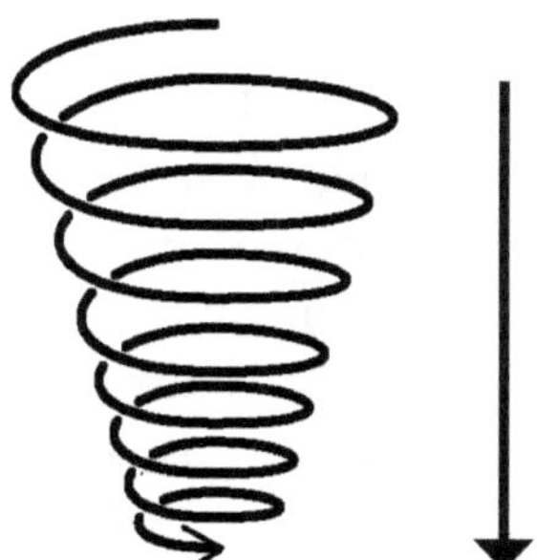

Isolation coupled with a negative thought pattern will always produce a self-consuming, ever-deepening downward spiral.

This is why we need other people. They may not understand, and if they have not been involved with depression or mental illness in any way, they will probably *not* understand, but it's okay. There are people who do understand and who have lived it, and some are privileged enough to be able to stand on the other side beyond it.

In marriages, I have watched men and women cut themselves off from their partners, the very people who love them the most and want to help them.

In the workplace I have seen people go so inward that they are beyond reach from others who genuinely desire to help. This can result in increased stress leave, sick leave, and absenteeism, loss of production and eventually loss of work. Following this, in many cases, the person suffering from depression or mental illness becomes a long-term unemployed person, which has such a crushing effect on them that they come to believe that they can never get beyond where they are and who they have become. There is a great need to break the cycle. To choose to bring those thoughts into captivity is vital, and consciously choosing to be around and open up to the right people is imperative to our healing.

In my case, I can honestly say to you today that I could not have made it without Robyn. I cannot over estimate the importance of this lady in my recovery. Every time I was down and heading lower and lower (some would say deeper and deeper into my cave) she had this amazing ability to get me out of it.

The crazy thing about Robyn is that she didn't really understand where my mind was taking me. She had not suffered from plummeting depressive episodes or mental illness, and could not fathom the depths I was plunging into. But her love for me would reach into my life and together we could walk though things. I learned that I had to let her in and not play games anymore. It was my choice to be totally open and vulnerable with her. In Australia we have what can be called a 'bloke thing' or you may call it the 'male thing'. It's all this 'real men don't cry' stuff. 'I'm a man and I will not show any weakness.'

Yet in our country, we have males between the age of 20 and 30 killing themselves at alarming rates. We have farmers who have fallen on hard times taking their own lives in large numbers because of so much hardship. This is a cultural flaw within our society. Real men do open up to people who care for them, and it literally saves lives!

Here is how it would play out between Robyn and me. Something would trigger my mind and it would start to run and over and over it would go. All of a sudden I would be heading down again. Robyn, with her female intuition, would say something like, "What's wrong honey?"

"Nothin," would be my very articulate reply.

"What's wrong, honey?"

"Nothin."

"What's wrong, honey?"

"Nothin."

(I could fill 300 pages just repeating this line, but I think you get the point).

She would wear me down. This woman you gave me, Lord, would wear me down. Now I could have stopped her and cut myself off, thinking that she would not understand, and I would have been right about her lack of understanding. What made the difference was not whether or not she could understand, but rather that she loved me enough to keep asking. If we don't open up, how can someone help?

SOME THINGS MAKE GOOD SENSE

There are some things that, over the years, you look back on and say, "Hey, that made sense," and you didn't even realize it at the time. As a couple we have always gone to bed at the same time. Even if one of us is reading after the other goes to sleep, we have always done this. It has been a great thing in our lives, as we spend great times of just simply discussing things together.

Can I give some marital advice here? I'm going to anyway. If you're a married person, try going to bed at the same time as your spouse. There are so many benefits—not just regarding mental health. Be open and talk if you need to. There is a very good chance that the person next to you is the one who cares more for you than anyone else on the planet.

MEN AND ISOLATION

I know men and women process issues differently. Men generally internalize what women externalize. I'm generalizing here, okay? Men internalize, we go into our 'cave' and we shut ourselves off. Why do men shut themselves off? The answer lies, in part, in our design as men. We are geared to fix things. Even hardware-challenged men like me are geared to fix things. We are geared to conquer and overcome and to win in life. We are designed as warriors. It's how God designed us and although it can drive the women in our lives a little crazy at times, it actually is a very good thing.

My girls are in general not very sporty. Some of them certainly could be, but music has won over their passion. I remember the school sports carnivals when my girls were little. Laura, my eldest, at age about seven or eight, would start the 50-meter sprint. I was on the sidelines yelling, "Come on, Laura! Come on, Laura!" and being the competitive dad. She would be going well until her friend next to her slowed up and then Laura would slow with her. What? Even worse, they would start to carry on a conversation as they sort of trotted the rest of the way, not even caring who won.

This throws the male mind into melt down. Come on, at least

try to win! You can talk after the race. A male is geared to win, or die in the effort. A male is geared to sacrifice for a cause greater than themselves, to conquer against great odds and opposition. It's what we do and it's a great thing, however, there are issues when a man cannot fix a situation or doesn't know how to. He is in a situation and cannot see a way out or any hope in the future. This is the most frightening place for a man. It is there that we tend to withdraw and close ourselves off. It is a coping mechanism that can help at times, but which, if left unchecked, will cause us to head deeper and deeper into ourselves until we cannot get ourselves out.

It is a frightening thing for a man to be in a place where he cannot see a way through whatever it is that is upon him.

This is why we love movies where the hero, against all odds, fights his way through 2,000 enemy troops single-handedly, crosses swollen rivers and climbs mighty mountains without ropes, clinging to cliff faces by his teeth while fighting off enemy gunships with a pocket knife. A man watching identifies with the hero. In reality though, he might be a father with massive responsibilities and feeling stuck without hope for the future. Is it any wonder we have men walking out on relationships at alarming rates? Men self-medicate with drug usage to escape, and I include the most common drug of all in our society, alcohol.

Take this situation. A man finds himself suffering with depression. He knows there is an issue yet will not talk about it. What was at first a case of low grade depression becomes deeper as he becomes more consumed by his thoughts. As thoughts do, they lead us deeper into more introspection, yet without a solution, the thoughts become a cage of negativity, deeper each day until everything that happens in that man's life reinforces his thoughts. This adds to their consuming nature until he starts to believe the ultimate lie—that he will never be able to move beyond this situation, that he is useless because he cannot fix it and that there is no hope. He begins to close himself off. He is a man lost in himself, consumed by thought and suffering with illness. If not interrupted by hope, this can, and sadly does, lead in many cases, to suicide or mental breakdown.

Wouldn't it be fantastic if help was sought at an early stage? To reach out and get help early can literally save your life and the life of your family. If this is speaking to you today, and you are in those first stages of this rather sad scenario, reach out and seek help. I had to ask myself some serious questions while in the process of writing of this book. One of the questions was what I wanted for the reader out of it? I came up with this answer. If just one person reading these pages sees that they are in trouble and gets in touch with someone who can help; if one life is saved by the hope presented in this book, then for all eternity I will sing for joy. I've walked this road and, in many cases, learned some of these lessons the hard way. It's my hope that you will not have to go through some of the stuff I did. It is my hope that what took me 20 years to reach, I can impart to you and help *you* get there in a lot shorter time.

Come on men. There is a chance of victory, yes the odds may be stacked against us, and yes the enemy seems to have greater forces. But isn't this why we have been created? There is hope and a brighter future. There is victory no matter how long and hard the road may be.

POWER OF ASSOCIATION

Never underestimate the importance of having the right people around you!

It's called the power of association. Someone once said, "If you want to know what you will be like in five years, look at the people you are hanging around now, and the books you are reading." This is so true and the reality is that if in my life I hang around liars, I will probably become a liar. If I hang around alcoholics, I will probably become an alcoholic. For years, people have tried to blame drinking problems solely on DNA, saying it is the reason why children who grow up with an alcoholic parent generally follow and become addicted to alcohol. I'm not saying that there may not be some kind of natural weakness. What I am saying is that it's far more to do with the fact that the alcoholic parents have taught the next generation a coping mechanism for difficulties. It is so much more a learned behavior than a function of DNA. This is the same for abusive relationships and deceitful situations.

This power of association can be both negative and positive. Make no mistake, there are times when we have to stand back and look at those we spend time with and ask a serious question. Are these people helping me or hindering me?

I've noticed that when a sufferer of depression or mental illness cuts themselves off from a positive environment, they still crave connection with people but generally choose to surround themselves with negative associations, thinking these people understand and can help—but they don't help at all! As well-meaning as these associations may be, they actually only serve to reinforce the negative and accelerate the downward spiral within our minds.

The power of getting around the right people is huge. The power of reading a good positive book over spending time in front of daytime television or teen soap operas cannot be overestimated.

The Bible tells us this:

1 Corinthians 15:33

Do not be misled: 'bad company corrupts good character.'

1 Corinthians 15:33 (NLT)

Don't be fooled by those who say such things, for 'bad company corrupts good character'.

What does this mean? It means we can stop kidding ourselves. If we are around negative people who pull us down we will be corrupted by them. Simply put, the wrong people can mess us up big time. The word in the passage for 'bad' or 'evil' is the word *kakos,* meaning 'of a bad nature and not as it ought to be'. Also, this relates to thinking, feeling and acting. Sometimes we have to choose. Do I continue along the same road that I have always walked and not get better, or do I choose a different road and change? One of the things I love most about the Bible is the positive nature of what it says and the overriding positive message of a better day and better hope and that tomorrow can be ours if we better position ourselves.

God's truths teach us to position ourselves around people who can help us and, within this, trust His wisdom and not pull back and isolate ourselves. *'He who walks with the wise grows wise.'* **Proverbs 13:20**

He even says:

Psalm 68:6

God sets the lonely in families.

Galatians 6:2

Bear one another's burdens and so fulfill the law of Christ.

Romans 12:15

Mourn with those who mourn.

FAMILY

The family God brings us into is His family. It's not perfect, but what family is? I have seen stuff that disgusts me within the church, yet I have forged, through many trials, some of the greatest friends you could ever imagine—people who have lifted me when I have fallen, warmed me when I was cold and stood beside me in the heat of battle. When I talk about the church, I'm not talking about some stuffy dead organization, but rather a positive, vibrant, life-filled organism. A place where it's real. Real people loving God in a real way. Authentic Christ-following people with a passionate love for life and others. When it comes to not trying to do this thing alone, it's not a religious organization that will make the difference, it's people!

A NOTE REGARDING CHURCHES

I think at times we expect too much of the church. God is perfect and for some reason we seem to expect that people in the church should be also. It is simply a false idea of what the church is. What is the church? Fundamentally, it is a group of people from all walks of life and all socio-economic levels who are all at various stages of their journey and who all are battling with something at any given time, coming together to love God and each other.

There is, in western society, the emergence of the mega-church culture and even, what some would call experience-based Christianity. This can lead to a situation of impersonal church attendance. This is true; however, in defense of the larger or even mega-church set up, they do a huge amount of work to connect people at a home base level. This is entirely scriptural, as in the start of the New Testament church the people met in houses, sat together and broke bread in their houses.

In a large church, these smaller groups that meet in houses or cafés are where so much of the great work for the Kingdom of God takes place. These are areas where friendships are forged and relationships built. These are the groups of people that are perfect for someone suffering with depression or mental illness to come into and simply be real with. It takes trust on both sides. It takes a willingness to be open and vulnerable. I know that it is a step of faith to enter in to these places, but here again, it's our choice what we do.

In our church, we call our small groups 'life groups', as many other churches do. Why? Because we do life together. It is in these places where we can be ourselves. I've had people come to church, who then leave and say totally stupid things like, "Everyone's so perfect in your church, and I'm so messed up. I just don't fit in." I understand this thinking, and in fact, I have thought it myself. However, it simply is not true. Of course everybody puts on their best for a Sunday service. It's a celebration. Yet it's in these smaller life groups that we build the great relationships that will be the difference in the end.

Friendships take time, but they are worth every second. I love Sunday services, but in all honesty I would much rather people be involved in small groups than Sunday meetings.

There is a passage in the Old Testament that illustrates the importance of friendship well.

Exodus 17:8-13

The Amalekites came and attacked the Israelites at Rephidim. Moses said to Joshua, 'choose some of our men and go out to fight the Amalekites. Tomorrow I will stand on top of the hill with the staff of God in my hands.'

So Joshua fought the Amalekites as Moses had ordered, and Moses, Aaron and Hur went to the top of the hill. As long as Moses held up his hands, the Israelites were winning, but whenever he lowered his hands, the Amalekites were winning.

When Moses' hands grew tired, they took a stone and put it under him and he sat on it. Aaron and Hur held his hands up—one on one side, one on the other—so that his hands remained steady until sunset. So Joshua overcame the Amalekite army with the sword.

Think of Aaron and Hur. There they are on top of the hill holding Moses' hands up when the heat of the day caused him to grow weary. Picture Moses: he could see that the battle was altered by his actions; he knew that friends died when he lowered his hands. There was plenty of motivation and willpower to keep his hands up. His love for God was great and his passion for God's people was equally as great, yet with all the good intentions, plans, understanding and passion, he still suffered from the weariness of being human and his hands began to fall. I wonder what he thought as his strength was leaving him? 'I cannot do it anymore. I have failed. Hurry up and kill the rest of those rotten Amalekites so I can get a coffee at Gloria Jean's before it closes.' I don't know, but I do know this. The battle would have been lost if it had not been for two men who stood beside another man and held up his arms when his strength was spent.

Read this next verse and I want you grab something here:

Matthew 18:20 (NASB)

"For where two or three have gathered together in My name, I am there in their midst."

Think about this. This section talks about when two or three gather in His name then God is in the midst on them.

This is the most quoted verse in opening prayers of small churches when the numbers are down a little. Come on, it's true, I've been there. Let's take it out of the church 'meeting on Sunday' setting. Put this verse into whenever anyone, and for the sake of the purpose for this book, someone who is suffering with depression or mental illness meets with another person. They meet together and although it may be tentative and perhaps just a light conversation over a coffee, two are gathering and believe it or not, God is in the mix. I know the theology that the presence of God is with a believer at all times and that we are never alone with Christ. He is not only with us, but in us. These things are true; however, what I believe God is trying to get across to us through this passage, amongst other things, is that there is eternal power at work within these meetings. In these friendships, God is there.

GOD IS IN THE MIX

When it comes to small groups of believers being together and friendships being forged, God is in the mix. Help is given, God is in the mix. People being vulnerable with one another, God is in the mix. You come to my house and we spend time just discussing things, God is in the mix. And when I hold your hands up, or you hold my hands up, we are still connecting with each other to help bring about the victory that needs to be won. God is in the mix.

GOD IS INFUSED INTO THESE GATHERINGS

Simply put, when I get help for depression, whether it be from a Christian counselor, doctor, ministry team member and or a friend, in the decision to work through this thing called mental illness, God is there as part of that choice, witnessing and helping by His spirit to bring a person beyond depression and mental illness, no matter how long it takes.

Here we can see the 'threefold cord' at work again. It is not easily broken, and I will tell you that if you have suffered long-term depression or mental illness, these fortified strongholds that you are choosing to stand against will not be easily broken. But broken down they can and must be!

1 Corinthians 3:9

For we are God's fellow workers; you are God's field, God's building.

We read in 1 Corinthians 12:12-27 about the body having many parts. So in the light that we are meant to be part of a body, or large group of parts, when we read something like, '*It is not good for man to be alone'* (**Genesis 2:18**), we can see clearly that God intended all along for us to be with other people. Seeing that it is clear that we need other people around us, let us spend some time thinking about an even greater need we have.

I COULD NEVER HAVE MADE IT WITHOUT HIM.

Psalm 145:14 (NLT)

The Lord helps the fallen and lifts those bent beneath their loads.

Psalm 145:14 (MSG)

God gives a hand to those down on their luck, gives a fresh start to those ready to quit.

We could read the entire 'self-help' book range at the local supplier, and there are myriads of them but sometimes we don't need self-help, because that is generally what got us into the mess. We need God-help! God has been my help in time of need, my comforter and my counselor, my truest friend and greatest companion.

This is huge. I have found him faithful!

I can stand here as one who is living life beyond the grip of depression and mental illness. The fog has lifted, the sun is shining and I can say that God has proven Himself to be faithful.

All my life I felt like I was walking on the edge of a knife and at any moment I would fall. In fact, I felt it was only a matter of time. But not anymore! My feet will not slip because He holds me secure. The Bible tells me that nothing can pluck me from His hand. Neither height nor depth. Those depths I know—and I know He walks with me and rescues me from sinking into darkness. The Bible puts it this way: 'nor depth'.

Romans 8:37-39 (NLT)

No, despite all these things, overwhelming victory is ours through Christ, who loved us.

And I am convinced that nothing can ever separate us from God's love. Neither death nor life, neither angels nor demons, neither our fears for today nor our worries about tomorrow—not even the powers of hell can separate us from God's love. No power in the sky above or in the earth below—indeed, nothing in all creation will ever be able to separate us from the love of God that is revealed in Christ Jesus our Lord.

Romans 8:39

Neither height nor depth, nor anything else in all creation, will be able to separate us from the love of God that is in Christ Jesus our Lord.

The importance of firstly knowing Christ, then understanding that the nature of God is to help us through our issues so that we become what he has always destined us to become, is vital to recovery.

Luke 10:27

"Love the Lord your God with all your heart, soul, mind and strength."

Do you need a new start today? If you regard yourself as a Christian, and if God has touched you through these pages, then you know you need His help. Now is your time. Today is the day. It truly is the first day of the rest of our lives. The question is where we live the rest of our lives and how we choose to live it. You may have said you are a Christian and prayed a prayer sometime and genuinely meant it, yet time and circumstances have taken you into the darkness of depression and mental illness. Is it your time to start a fresh life? Be prepared that you may still suffer mentally for a time. Emotions will still get confused, but gradually over time, doing and understanding these principles, your sickness will be healed and you will reach beyond the illness.

PRAY WITH ME.

Heavenly Father, I thank You for Your loving kindness that draws me ever closer to You.

I have wandered, and for this I am truly sorry.

I have trusted my thoughts over Your word, God, please forgive me for this and help me trust You more.

Today, I choose to leave the past behind me and to walk in the newness of life given by You, Lord.

I choose today, to own where I am and who I have become and look to You, Lord, for my future. I offer You all of me; my heart, my soul and especially my mind and my strength.

Make me new, Lord.

You forgive and cleanse fully, and as Your word declares: 'though my sins were as scarlet they will be whiter than snow.'

Today I choose to forgive, as I have been forgiven.

To let go of the pain and heartaches.

Today I simply lay them at Your feet, Lord, and cast all my cares upon You, because You care for me.

Thank you for Your forgiveness and love.

Now take my life, and let it be fully Yours from this day forth; in Jesus' name I ask this,

Amen.

FIRST TIMERS

This may be the first time you have really understood the love of God for you. So here is what needs to be done. You need to openly pray a prayer to God. There is no set formula for this prayer, except that it does involve elements of thankfulness, repentance or sorrow for the things we have done, a turning from them, and an offering of our lives to Christ, with a determination to follow Him from this day forward. I have put a suggested prayer below, however, if you would like to add more, then go for it. This is a direct conversation between you and your creator. Make it as personal as you can because God is very close to you right now, and will hear every word you pray.

Today I see a hope in You, God.

Today I choose to step into the light.

Today I ask for forgiveness for all I have done wrong. Please help me forgive others as now You have forgiven me.

Thank you for loving someone like me, Lord.

I give you my past, my today and my future.

I lay down all my hurts before You, Lord.

I give you my habits, and if they are bad, I thank you in advance for the power to change.

Today I give You my heart, my soul, my mind and my strength.

I choose, from this day forward, to entrust my life to the living God.

Let Your strength be made known through my weakness.

Let my life, from this day forward, bring honor and glory to you God.

Amen.

Congratulations. You have just started a new life, angels are partying and I am so proud of you.

WHAT TO DO NOW

It is ridiculous to think that with a simple prayer we will have a dramatic and permanent change if we don't allow change in our behavior. A person coming off alcohol, for instance, needs to put strategies in place to avoid the temptations of alcohol getting a grip on their lives again. So here are five strategies to put in place that will have a great positive effect on our lives from this day forward.

1. LOVE GOD AND OTHER PEOPLE

Matthew 22:36-40

'Teacher, which is the greatest commandment in the Law?' Jesus replied: 'Love the Lord your God with all your heart and with all your soul and with all your mind'. This is the first and greatest commandment. And the second is like it: 'Love your neighbor as yourself'. All the Law and the Prophets hang on these two commandments.

Determining to love God with your entire life, heart, soul, mind and strength and choosing to love others will be vital to continued recovery. It never stops amazing me how simply choosing to love others and thinking about them rather than ourselves can change our entire perspective on life and result in true happiness being birthed in our lives.

2. GET THE WORD OF GOD INTO YOU

This is the same advice that an old man gave me when I first started on this journey: "Get the word of God into you, read big chunks of it." Start at the gospel of John or Mark. There is probably nothing that will change your life more positively than an effective Bible reading time.

3. PRAYER TO GOD

Prayer is a direct communication with God. It is simply talking and listening to God as you would to a friend. Be honest with Him, you won't offend Him. Cry, sing, shout, yell, stand up, sit, and kneel. Just be real! God is with you right now, and a conversation is not some religious duty to be performed in a strict type of pattern. It is simply a conversation as you would have with a very close friend.

Philippians 4:6-7

Do not be anxious about anything, but in everything, by prayer and petition, with thanksgiving, present your requests to God. And the peace of God, which transcends all understanding, will guard your hearts and your minds in Christ Jesus.

4. GO TO A CHURCH OR SMALL GROUP

Get connected with other people. We cannot do this thing alone. It is vital, as we have just gone through in the chapter, that we be connected. Learn to worship God for His greatness. If your church group cannot offer you this connection, then find one that will. Get connected to people!

5. TELL OTHERS ABOUT THIS GREAT HOPE

If you are serious about the prayers you have just prayed, then tell someone what you've done. Not in some hyper-faith, 'I've prayed a prayer and everything's fixed way' but just simply telling someone about the journey you're on and the direction you have chosen to walk. If that prayer was the first time you've ever prayed to God and you have asked Jesus into your life, then it's a great time to celebrate a new beginning. All the angels in heaven are celebrating right now over what you have done. Understand this, there is noone more excited than God Himself because one of His lost children has decided to come home.

Mark 16:15 (NLT)

And then he told them, "Go into all the world and preach the Good News to everyone".

God is going to start to do major changes in your life. This passage below describes what He has done for me, and what He will do for you;

Isaiah 61:3

...And provide for those who grieve in Zion—to bestow on them a crown of beauty instead of ashes, the oil of gladness instead of mourning, and a garment of praise instead of a spirit of despair. They will be called oaks of righteousness, a planting of the LORD for the display of his splendor.

I know without doubt that the most important reason I can even write these pages has been the miraculous power of God. He has turned my darkness into light, my hatred into happiness and my pain into peace. '*In Him I live and move and have my being.*' **Acts 17:28**

I see, and I have beauty now instead of ashes, and happiness instead of sorrow.

MAKINGLIFEABETTERPLACETOLIVE

A PERSONAL LETTER

So there it is. You have my story and the nine steps toward recovery. I hope you have been able to identify and learn a few things as we have traveled together for this time, and also that I have, in some way, been able to equip you for this journey. I encourage you to be particular and determined about applying these principles to your life. As arctic explorers and mountaineers know, the right equipment is the difference between life and death. So they are meticulous, if not fastidious, regarding their equipment. I know the equipment laid out before you in these chapters will not fail you.

I sincerely hope my heart has come through these pages. In life's journeys, it will get cold and the wind will be outside your tent threatening with gale force to blow you to oblivion. The right equipment will hold. These principles are firm and secure. They will anchor you in the storms and equip you to climb. They will guide you through blizzards and help you cross raging waters. When the sky darkens, they will be a light to you and a lamp to guide your steps.

THISHAPPENED,THATTHEGREATNESSOFGODMIGHTBE DISPLAYED

As we draw to a close of this book, let's examine one more biblical story together. This fascinating true story appears in chapter 9 of John's gospel. It's called the healing of the man born blind.

The concept put forward here is so foreign to our western society. It's the concept that suffering is indeed something that God has destined to bring glory to Himself. I guess it probably shouldn't be that hard to comprehend, as Jesus Himself suffered so much for us to bring glory to the Father. In the passage below we see Jesus' disciples walking with Jesus and asking questions. Observe the question they ask, as we consider the questions we at times ask, and the answer Jesus gave to them. We always ask and reason from our past experience and preconceived ideas. Jesus blows this thinking away through this passage.

John 9:1-7 (MSG)

Walking down the street, Jesus saw a man blind from birth. His disciples asked, 'Rabbi, who sinned: this man or his parents, causing him to be born blind?' Jesus said, "You're asking the wrong question. You're looking for someone to blame. There is no such cause-effect here. Look instead for what God can do....".

He said this and then spit in the dust, made a clay paste with the saliva, rubbed the paste on the blind man's eyes, and said, "Go, wash at the Pool of Siloam" (Siloam means 'sent'). The man went and washed—and saw.

This story goes on for the whole of John chapter 9 and the healing causes a great uproar amongst the religious leaders of the day. Jesus goes on to show the difference between natural blindness and true blindness in a spiritual realm.

Let us just grab a single truth from this passage as an illustration of how we should approach depression and mental illness and the long and difficult road to recovery. Don't we ask similar questions at times; 'who caused this depression or mental illness—was it parents, family, work, natural weakness, substance abuse?'

Imagine this man who was born blind. He was born with a

physical weakness—a lack of sight. It was not the result of sinful behavior of his parents. He was simply born blind. Somewhere in the mix of his DNA his sight had been lost. Now this man had been blind for a long time. In fact, he had been with this condition for all his life—blind for over 40 years. Darkness had shrouded him all his days. Through no fault of his own or anyone else he had suffered for over 40 years. His life was ruled by a weakness within him that he neither caused nor could fix.

Then Jesus comes along, spits in the mud, and makes a mud pie. He slaps the pie on the man's face and tells him to find his own way to a pool and wash it off. Thank you very much Jesus. There was no, "Hey John, take this man to the pool." Just, "go on, walk in what I tell you to do, and you will see."

Imagine this blind man heading toward the pool and people saying, "Look at him," "What happened to you, man?" There was mud dripping off his face as he stumbled along. Someone may have quipped, "Who would do that to a poor blind man?" But he stepped in his blindness toward the water. He still could not see while he walked but he walked and stumbled on, not giving up, not sitting back down to beg, not complaining about the saliva and mud dripping down his face. He just kept walking. He went where he was sent and he did what was asked of him, then *bam!* He could see.

Even if you, at this stage, cannot see clearly and the mud seems to cover your eyes, don't worry. The mud just shows that Jesus has already touched you and you are in the process of recovery. Just keep stepping forward, one step after the other. Yes, there may be a stumble, but just keep going and you will see.

Let's go back to the conversation between the disciples and Jesus, ask the question regarding *our* lives, and see what Jesus just might say about us. We, like the disciples, can be asking the wrong question simply because as humans we are bred to recognize cause and effect. That way, there is always something or someone to blame and a reason for the predicaments we find ourselves in. Let us turn our eyes and ears to what Jesus said:

John 9:2-3 (MSG)

His disciples asked, 'Rabbi, who sinned: this man or his parents, causing him to be born blind?' Jesus said, "You're asking the wrong question. You're looking for someone to blame. There is no such cause-effect here. Look instead for what God can do".

'Look instead for what God can do.'

Let this be an anthem for our lives from this point on: "Look instead for what God can do". The New International Version puts it this way: 'This happened that the work of God might be displayed in his life.'

What if we are asking the wrong question? What if whatever you or I have been through, and where you are today, is not to be looked at as a question of blame, but rather from the perspective of what God can do. The perspective that says, 'This happened that the work of God might be displayed in his (or her) life.' I believe this to be so because I have lived to see it in my own life. Jesus came walking along and even while all my questioning about 'why this, and why that' was not answered, Jesus said: *'It's okay, son, all this happened so that the work of God might be displayed in your life.'*

It's not to condone the past or destructive influences, but rather to say, "All our lives from this day forward, can be to show the works of God's might."

We can see that in Bible times, blindness had a stigma of guilt and shame, due to the disciples reasoning about who was guilty to bring this situation on him. Depression or mental illness is like that in our society today, with the stigma and associated guilt and shame. Instead, let us look with our lives to what God can do! We will see!

I have learned that God is not distant and that even in the

darkest of times, He is there; that when I think the blackness will hide me, even blackness is as light to Him. This is brilliant: the Bible says, '*What is man that you are mindful of him.*' **Psalm 8:4** We are but specks on this terrestrial ball, floating in the midst of the endless universe. Earth is a little blue dot against the vastness of space. Yet, the creator of all the wonders of this incredible universe is mindful of us. He chooses to love and live amongst us. He chooses to take our weaknesses and use them for the glory of God and a better life for us.

We could ask the questions, "why did Jesus wait 40 years to heal this man? Why did he let him suffer so much?" I certainly would love to ask about the whole spitting and mud pie thing—how weird is that? It does, however, prove that God works in unexpected ways at times and certainly does not work the same way every time. It is so easy to get into the 'what if', 'if only' or, 'I should have' mindsets, and spend our lives living in regret and the past. We cannot change one second of our past, but we certainly can take steps to alter our future. We are who we are right now. Let us make choices not from the past and its inevitable regrets but rather make choices today based on looking for what God can do.

Remember we looked at those verses in Ecclesiastes 3:11. To refresh our memories here is the verse again.

Ecclesiastes 3:11

He has made everything beautiful in its time. He has also set eternity in the hearts of men; yet they cannot fathom what God has done from beginning to end.

I am sure the blind man looked anything but beautiful as he walked toward the pool with the whole mud and saliva thing happening all over his face. Yet, through those steps he was healed. He became beautiful because there is nothing more beautiful than a person changed by the power of God.

'He has made everything beautiful in its time' is one of the greatest statements for us to grab and hold onto. The verse also says, 'Yet they cannot fathom what God has done from beginning to end.' Our lives are not at an end yet. We are still moving through and we cannot fathom His hands' work from beginning to end. I am believing and hoping with all my heart that although we cannot fully understand God's working, we will choose to trust *in* His working. The stability we gain from this will be huge. The following few verses have had a significant impact on my life.

Psalm 37:31

The law of his God is in his heart; his feet do not slip.

Psalm 40:1-2

I waited patiently for the LORD; he turned to me and heard my cry.

He lifted me out of the slimy pit, out of the mud and mire; he set my feet on a rock and gave me a firm place to stand.

Psalm 55:22 (NLT)

Give your burdens to the LORD and he will take care of you. He will not permit the godly to slip and fall.

I do not claim to be a scholar or even a learned man. All I know is that there is hope for a better life—a life free from the cage of our minds. I know it not because anyone has told me, or because it is written in a book. I know it because I have lived it. I have lived, and almost died, within my mind, and yes, I still remember the pain of mental illness. However, I know what it is like to be able to live a productive, wonderful life beyond the confines of depression and mental illness. Your journey may be one of three steps forward and two steps back, but keep on stepping forward. It will not be an easy road. I hope I have not given that impression, but keep stepping anyway. Sometimes taking the right road means we travel up a steep hill.

All I know is: it is worth every step of the journey! I can

honestly say today that my life is so much better for the taking of the journey.

Each of these steps will involve challenges and at times pain, but keep stepping! The high mountain pass awaits you, the climb will be steep at times, the exposure great, and it will seem to zig and zag back and forth as you go, but don't give up—keep stepping forward.

Keep going, step after step, and when you reach the top, the fog will have cleared and the sun will be shining. I look forward to you standing alongside me, for the view truly is spectacular!

Many thanks,

Gary

ABOUT GARY BLACKFORD

I have been on an incredible journey. My journey, like all journeys has had some high mountain top experiences and some deep, cold and very dark valleys as well. I used to think I was alone in my suffering, but now I know that so many live where I once lived, and this book is designed to help lead as many as possible to a life beyond depression and mental illness. Although born in country New South Wales, I spent most my younger years in Sydney, Australia, during the 70's and 80's. Around the age of 16-17, life shifted and I began walking a road that would lead me to darker places than I ever imagined existed in my mind. Hallucinations, paranoia, paralysing fear and depression became constant companions, an all consuming blackness that culminated in a suicide attempt in 1986. Now I am a Senior Pastor, biblical teacher, professional sales and business development trainer, winner of numerous awards for sales and account development, and have established a successful small business, I speak and running training seminars in various fields. I love life, live and pastor in Coffs Harbour NSW Australia. I enjoy being married to my wife Robyn and have for 20+ years, I also father 4 amazing daughters. How did all this happen? Enjoy the read!

Thanks for picking up my book, I hope it has a powerful affect in your life.

Gary

www.ingramcontent.com/pod-product-compliance
Lightning Source LLC
LaVergne TN
LVHW010055110826
845155LV00028B/352

* 9 7 8 1 9 2 1 5 8 9 7 2 0 *